PENGU

THE JUN

Judith Wills is one of Britain's leading slimming experts. She has been the freelance Editor of the popular diet magazine *Slimmer* for several years. She has written regularly on slimming, healthy eating, fitness and related topics for various national newspapers and magazines over the past twelve years — including the *Daily Mail*, *Daily Star*, *Sunday People*, *Prima*, *Woman* and *Woman and Home* — and has broadcast on local radio all over the UK. She has built up a strong reputation for giving sensible, practical advice and is definitely against all 'cranky' and extreme eating habits and dieting methods. Judith Wills lives in Herefordshire with her husband, Tony Allen, and their two children, William and Christopher. She wrote *The Junk Food Diet* after Christopher's birth, when she lost nearly a stone following its principles.

Judith Wills

THE JUNK FOOD DIET

SLIM ON THE FOOD
YOU LIKE

Penguin Books

For my family

PENGUIN BOOKS

Published by the Penguin Group
27 Wrights Lane, London W8 5TZ, England
Viking Penguin Inc., 40 West 23rd Street, New York, New York 10010, USA
Penguin Books Australia Ltd, Ringwood, Victoria, Australia
Penguin Books Canada Ltd, 2801 John Street, Markham, Ontario, Canada L3R 1B4
Penguin Books (NZ) Ltd, 182–190 Wairau Road, Auckland 10, New Zealand

Penguin Books Ltd, Registered Offices: Harmondsworth, Middlesex, England

First published 1989
1 3 5 7 9 10 8 6 4 2

Filmset in Monophoto 10 on 12pt Melior

Made and printed in Great Britain by
Richard Clay Ltd, Bungay, Suffolk

ACKNOWLEDGEMENTS

Very special thanks to the many people who helped make this book possible: my husband, Tony, for putting up with it – and me – and for all that research; Jane Turnbull for her much needed encouragement and faith; Pamela Dix for sorting everything out so professionally; and Eleanor, Sally, Janette and Lesley for their constructive criticism.

The Junk Food Diet has been medically approved by Dr Eleanor Clarke, a GP and mother with a special interest in women's health and obesity, and has been nutritionally approved by Dr Sally Parsonage, a State Registered Dietician and author of several publications on family nutrition.

J. W.
October 1988

CONTENTS

down or stops . . . what to do if you lose weight too quickly . . . diet tips and rules . . . list of unlimited food items throughout the diet.

intake with anyone else's ... how to build up your calorie level gradually ... your maintenance diet ... eating and lifestyle tips ... what to do should the unthinkable happen! ... learning to be a slim person ... three simple stages to beat binges for ever.

How kids' nutrition needs differ from adults' ... how many of the foods kids love are good for them! ... why there is no need to ban sweet foods from your child's diet ... the simple traffic light guide to a healthy 'junk' diet for your child ... junk food and the additives debate ... junk food and ability ... overweight children − how to slim them down painlessly ... height/weight chart for kids ... planning your child's menu.

How to use the recipe section ... succulent sauces ... super bread snacks ... tasty egg and cheese meals ... unboring fish meals ... chicken and turkey dishes ... pasta and rice dishes ... red meat dishes galore.

A unique directory of over 350 foods − everything from hot dogs to gateau as well as more basic foods − listing calories, protein, fat, fibre, calcium, iron, vitamin C and added-sugar content in an average portion.

INTRODUCTION

———

Junk food is fattening food.

If you really want to lose weight, you'll have to alter your diet radically.

The only way to slim is to become vegetarian.

Those are just some of the phrases you will have been hearing — until you're sick of them — over the past few years.

Now I'm blatantly and guiltlessly going to lead you into rebellion! Stick with me and I'll show you how you can slim, and stay healthy, on all the food you like — without ever having to eat a vegetable burger again!

It was perhaps inevitable that the slimming industry would jump on the 'healthy eating' bandwagon. What makes a healthy diet has been one of the big talking points of the 1980s. Guided by various trials and studies, culminating in the government's 1984 COMA report — whose main suggestion was that we should reduce our consumption of fat — self-appointed slimming gurus have virtually led us to believe that *all* foods containing animal fat — or, by the way, sugar, salt or additives, or without a large dose of bran — are akin to arsenic, and that to eat them and, heaven forbid, enjoy them is a sin!

Most of the famous diet books of the eighties have gone along with these ideas, recommending diets very low in (or free from) meat, high in raw foods, vegetables and fruit, packed full of fibre and vigorously avoiding anything processed.

Yes, the health food lobby *has* helped us greatly in leading to a more enlightened, balanced way of eating. But I am sure that a grossly limited diet is not the way to good health – or permanent slimness. There are millions of people in the Western world who have tried these 'new health' style diets and failed, long term, to lose weight on them, or, indeed, to become 'healthier'.

Were you one of them?

No wonder you couldn't follow the high fruit diet for long. It upset your stomach and made you light-headed. No wonder you didn't like the high-fibre diet. You couldn't put up with the flatulence and the bloating. No wonder you lost weight on the liquids-only diet, but put it all back on within weeks. It didn't help your day-to-day eating habits.

Limited-eating fad diets are definitely *not* what weight loss for life is all about. And they are not what you want.

What the famous slimming gurus forgot was that you can't change a nation's diet drastically and expect us all to adapt. It can't work for more than a while. That's why lost weight returns within a year for 80 per cent of dieters.

The foods we've been raised on must form a large part of any successful diet: meat, cheese, eggs, potatoes, bread. And so must all the foods that have, in the last twenty years or so, become an important part of our lives: the takeaways, the pizzas, the burgers, the kebabs.

These are all foods that have, in recent years, been saddled with the label 'junk'. They are the foods that we are now made to feel guilty about eating and enjoying.

And yet sales figures and my own surveys prove that these are the foods you *like* (even if they are no longer the foods you have the nerve to serve up when neighbours come to supper).

So, for a change, I've got some good news for you. I'm going to show you just why so-called 'junk' food isn't junk food at all, and that there is no such thing as a 'healthy' food – or, come to that, an 'unhealthy' one.

And I'm going to tell you how you can slim – and stay slim for life – on the food you *really like.*

Burgers, bangers, convenience meals, roast lamb, pork and beef, egg and chips, fish and chips, steak and chips, roast potatoes, baked potatoes, mashed potatoes, crisps, white bread, Indian takeaways, Chinese takeaways, pizza, doner kebabs, toast, bacon, fish fingers, chilli, spaghetti . . .

Are you beginning to like the sound of this? I've not finished! You can also slim – and stay slim – without having to give up the treats you like best: chocolate, ice cream, biscuits, cakes, desserts, cheesecake, even alcohol. In fact, all the things you thought you could never eat on a slimming diet – let alone a healthy one!

Even better, I'm going to show you how you need not – unless you want to – eat vegetarian meals, grapefruit, lentils, cottage cheese, boiled greens, brown rice, steamed fish, crispbreads, celery, or lettuce ever again!

On my Junk Food Diet you will slim easily because you won't feel deprived of your favourite foods – or anxious that you've got to grapple with a whole new style of eating. You needn't worry about how the family will react to different menus or, alternatively, have the bother of cooking separate meals for yourself. Everyone can follow this diet, whether or not they are slimming.

You need spend no extra money or go hunting for unusual ingredients. You need go near no health food shops or attempt to master vegetarian cookery. I'm going to show you how you can carry on shopping at your favourite supermarket or local store. And – most important – you needn't worry or feel guilty that in some way you are damaging your health by eating the foods you like.

The Junk Food Diet will show you how so-called junk

foods and everyday foods can be part of your regular eating pattern and still give you a diet well within those COMA eating guidelines (given in detail in Chapter 2).

The Junk Food Diet doesn't expect you to attempt the impossible. It does expect you to want to carry on with your normal life.

So, if you desperately want to slim and yet still be able to say yes to the supermarket, yes to family food, yes to takeaways, yes to ready meals, yes to cans and packets and jars, then here is your diet.

It's all you need to stay slim – and healthy – for life.

1 · THE CASE FOR JUNK FOOD

Every one of us has a 'health freak' acquaintance who piously raises an eyebrow at the sight of us tucking into chips or a steak or – heaven forbid – sliced white bread with real butter on it. 'How *can* you eat that junk?' they'll say.

Yet what is junk?

Long before burgers were invented 'junk' was the dry, salted meat that sailors ate on board ship when it was a choice between that or starvation. In the sixties and seventies junk became another word for fast food and sweet snacks. But in the eighties the word 'junk' has been used with greater and greater abandon. Some dictionaries describe it as 'food of poor nutritional quality' or 'food of little nutritional value'. These phrases are, of necessity, vague, because in the precise world of applied nutrition *there is no such thing as 'junk food'*! And when I began asking around for ordinary people's definition of junk, I began to understand why the dieticians don't use the word.

In my verbal poll I asked a wide cross-section of people from all incomes and age groups to say exactly what they would classify as junk food. The foods mentioned most often were these: sugary foods, chocolate, sweets, chips, takeaways, bought cakes, biscuits, fizzy drinks, instant mixes.

Not far behind were these: ice cream, tinned puddings, red meat, Cheddar cheese, pasta, white bread, white rice, cornflakes and other cereals, tinned fruit.

By this time I was beginning to feel surprised that so many people felt so many foods were junk. And as my questioning progressed, I became more and more surprised. Here are some other answers I got to the question 'What is your definition of junk food?': all packeted foods, all canned foods, all processed foods, all foods containing added sugar, all foods containing added salt, all foods containing additives of any kind, all freeze-dried foods, all foods with some of their natural fibre content removed, all farmed foods.

There's more. A few people even said, all cooked food, all food that has been altered in any way from its natural state.

I finished my little survey and looked at my lists. I got out my nutrition books and spent some long time searching for foods not on my list of 'junk'. Do you know what I ended up with? The only foods that no one at all mentioned as being junk were: fresh fruit, fresh, raw vegetables, fresh herbs, naturally-dried nuts, seeds, grains and pulses, and wild birds and game (tracked and killed yourself, of course). That was all that was left.

My survey proved what I had suspected – that although the 'healthy eating' movement of the last decade has undoubtedly done us in the Western world a great deal of good, it has also done us harm. It has made us feel guilty about enjoying a wide variety of foods that are certainly not 'of little nutritional value'. It has made us fearful of damaging our health by eating almost anything from bread to bacon. If we listen to the anti-junk food doom-merchants' advice and cut out most of the things we enjoy, I believe we will limit our diets to such an extent that for every twentieth-century ill we prevent, we'll cause a new one.

Let's return to that oh-so-short list of 'non-junk foods'.

Far from making up the perfect, healthy diet, they present certain problems.

First, it would be very difficult to get a healthy diet – one containing all the nutrients we need, long-term – from such a limited selection of foods. So many of us would become ill through 'deficiency diseases'.

Then, few of us could stick to such a diet for long in any case. Think about it. Could you live on raw fruit and vegetables, feed a family, socialize, travel, work and live happily on those foods – even for a few days? No. Neither could I. I wouldn't want to. And we don't have to.

The idea that only a chosen few foods aren't junk is plainly ridiculous. And it is a terrible shame that we have to feel guilty about eating the things we like best. For like them we do.

Detailed questionnaires filled in by readers of my own magazine, *Slimmer*, and a poll I conducted in a national newspaper read by 1½ million people have shown conclusively what foods we really like (see Table 1).

These conclusions are backed up by the government's National Food Survey and sales figures for foods such as crisps, chocolate and takeaways.

It is nonsense to suggest that all processed and packaged food is junk, nonsense to say that all food containing saturated fat, or salt, or sugar is junk, and nonsense for the health food faddists to expect us to give them up.

· *HEALTHY JUNK FOOD* ·

Let's take a closer look at some of the foods most frequently described as 'junk' and see what's really in them.

Takeaways

Takeaways can mean anything from a chop suey to a cheeseburger, so it's impossible to lump them all together in one nutritional bag. At worst they can be high in fat and salt and low in fibre and vitamins. But at best they can – and often are – good nutritional value. The Consumers' Association of the UK analysed takeaway meals in 1988 and came to the same conclusion. (For more information on takeaways, see Chapter 2.)

White bread

My junk food poll participants said bread is junk because 'It has no fibre and no goodness left in it.' In fact, white bread does still contain fibre. It also contains protein and iron, and, unlike wholemeal bread, is a good source of calcium. And it has virtually no sugar and very little fat.

Cheddar (and other hard cheeses)

Condemned because 'It's full of animal fat', Cheddar is high in protein and is one of our major sources of calcium – unlike the soft cheeses, such as cottage cheese.

Chips

'Fatty stodge', 'Nothing good in them', 'Full of saturated fat'. In fact, well-cooked chips fried in corn oil are full of vitamin C, have a reasonable amount of fibre and a lot of potassium. They contain little saturated fat.

Beefburger

'Red meat is bad for you.' The average well-grilled or fried and drained burger is a goldmine of protein, iron and B vitamins, plus, in the bun, all the same goodies you get in white bread. It is surprisingly low in fat.

Canned beans in tomato sauce

'Processed pap,' said one poll participant. Actually, baked beans are rich in iron and protein, contain lots of fibre and there are plenty of brands with reduced sugar and salt.

Rich fruit cake

'No goodness in cake'. Wrong. A slice of fruit cake will give you plenty of fibre, some protein and some iron. In fact, depending on the recipe, it will contain some of almost everything we need, except vitamin C!

Egg and bacon

'My wife forbids me to eat it because of all the fat.' What a shame. Trimmed bacon, grilled or fried until crisp, with an egg fried in corn oil and drained, with its high iron, B vitamins and protein content will set any husband (or wife) up for the day!

Are you feeling less guilty yet? All the foods above (and hundreds more like them) are far from being junk; they are high in 'nutritional value'. And if you like them, you'd be silly to banish them from your diet.

· HEALTH FOOD – BUT IS IT? ·

In just the same way that 'junk' foods are often condemned

without a fair trial, many foods are now being sold as 'health' foods when, in fact, they are no more healthy than the foods we eat as junk.

Here are just some of the so-called 'health foods' that may not be as healthy as they seem.

Muesli

'The healthiest breakfast you can eat,' said several people when I delved into their views on a healthy diet. 'High in fibre and full of natural goodness,' said someone else. And so original Swiss muesli was – yet many brands of muesli contain sugar as one of the prime ingredients. Ah, but brown sugar. That's no better for you than white. Just as many mueslis also contain lots of added salt. And to make matters worse, muesli is no higher in fibre than many other *low* health-profile breakfast cereals!

Cereal bars and 'health' bars

'Much better for you than chocolate or sweets'. Perhaps the original concept of high-fibre cereal bars was good, but nearly all now contain high levels of sugar or one of its close relatives, fructose and glucose. They also contain salt and vegetable fat (often of the saturated kind). I bought a carob-coated 'health' bar and the list of ingredients read: sugar, palm kernel and palm oil (saturated), skimmed milk powder, lingonberry, carob powder, maltodextrin (a form of carbohydrate), lecithin (an emulsifier) and salt.

Wholemeal bread

'Much better for you than white'. Wholemeal bread's 'plus' is that it contains more fibre than ordinary white bread.

White bread's 'plus' is that it contains more calcium than wholemeal. If you happen to be one of the increasing number of people trying to get more calcium into your diet, it could logically be argued that white bread is 'better for you' than wholemeal.

Honey

'Natural sweetness'. Natural sweetness is just another word for sugar, and there's precious little else in honey at all.

Fruit

'Fresh, natural, full of vitamins'. This is an extreme example, I know, and of course good-quality fresh fruit can't be called 'junk'. But go into any greengrocer's store at the wrong time of the week or the wrong week of the year and you are liable to end up with a piece of fruit that is neither fresh nor full of vitamins. Fruit stored too long, especially in warm, light conditions, like under a shop awning in summer, will have lost a lot, or even most, of its vitamin C before you eat it. Natural? How do you know it hasn't been sprayed with a variety of chemicals for pest and disease control? Could it have been irradiated?

And, to end up with:

Cabbage

Freshly picked and quickly eaten it's wonderful, but when stored, chopped, boiled then kept waiting for the eater it becomes a 'junk' food with precious little vitamin C left and no more fibre than a slice of white bread!

So, you see, things aren't always what they seem. In

Chapter 2 I'll be looking more closely at all the nutrients we need for good health, and how the Junk Food Diet provides them for you within government health guidelines.

But what I want you to begin to realize is that you don't have to feel guilty about liking burgers, fish fingers, Chinese takeaways, chips and sausages. You don't have to pretend to your friends, like a secret alcoholic, that you don't eat these things.

No food properly prepared and eaten within a varied diet is junk. Individual foods are not 'healthy' or 'unhealthy'. It is how those foods join together to make up your diet over the weeks that will decide whether you're as healthy through nutrition as you could be or not.

So, although there are no junk foods, there is a junk diet – an unbalanced, limited diet within which you're getting too much of certain nutrients and too few of others. What you *don't* want to do is eat one or two foods to the exclusion of most others, whether your favourite happens to be ice cream and milk shake – or oranges. You can end up with a junk diet just as easily through eating too many of the so-called 'healthy' foods as you can on chocolate and chips. For instance, let's imagine you decide to go on a 'health kick' and eat nothing but oranges. You'd very soon get bad stomach ache, and would have to spend most of your day in the bathroom. If you stuck the diet out for weeks, you might get kidney stones and ulcers. And then some deficiency diseases like anaemia and rickets. And then some more.

Of course you wouldn't be so silly, but the fact is that fad eating of any kind will eventually make you unhealthy, and will often make you fat.

So eat your favourite foods within a varied diet. Eat your chips twice a week or maybe even more often. Eat a chocolate bar or a couple of oranges every day, if that's what you really like. There is *plenty* of room in your diet for all the foods you love.

And don't worry — you don't need to be weighed down with a nutrition manual. The Junk Food Diet will show you how to eat, and slim, on your favourite foods — for life.

· HOW JUNK FOODS CAN HELP YOU SLIM ·

Okay, so now you're convinced that you can join me on this rebellious diet without ruining your health. But can you *really* lose weight on all those fattening foods you love?

Yes, you can!

Let's look at what you have to do to lose weight.

Fact one: You can't lose weight unless, over a period of time, you take in (in what you eat and drink) fewer calories than your body will use up in its normal energy requirements. If your body isn't getting the energy it needs from the food and drink you put into it, it will get energy instead from the stored fat supplies within your body. So — like magic — you will get thinner!

Fact two: There is no method of losing weight (apart from temporary fluid weight) that will really work apart from the above method. You can help the fat-burning process along by stepping up your exercise levels so you use more energy (see Chapter 5).

Fact three: The number of calories you can eat and still lose weight varies enormously. A normal daily calorie consumption for a woman of average weight and height to maintain her weight is around 2,150. For a man of average weight and height the figure is around 2,750. If you are overweight, you have probably been eating more than that amount. It doesn't have to be a lot more. In calorie terms, 1 lb of fat on your body equals 3,500 calories you ate or drank that you didn't need. So, for example, if you are a woman and you eat 2,500 calories a day when you really only need 2,150 a day, within ten days – *only* ten days – you will have eaten 3,500 (2,500 − 2,150 × 10) calories more than you need and you may have put on 1 lb in weight!

That extra 350 calories a day represents one small snack. So don't think you have to be a pig to get fat. You don't. Now let's look at it the other way. You want to lose weight because you've been eating a steady 2,500 calories a day and it's made you fat. If you drop down to 1,500 calories a day (far more than most low-calorie diets suggest), you will be giving yourself a daily calorie deficit of 1,000. Over a week that is 7,000. To lose a pound of fat you have to have a deficit of 3,500 calories, so eating as much as 1,500 calories a day, you'll lose 2 lbs a week. That's 104 lbs in a year. Enough for almost anyone, I'd guess!

Of course, there are some people who for various reasons will need to diet on less than 1,500 calories a day. Some lucky people (mostly men) will be able to diet on more than 1,500 calories a day. All I want to point out here is that you won't be going hungry on the Junk Food Diet, and once your calorie level for dieting is decided upon (which it will be in Chapter 6), you will still slim whether you eat your calorie allowance in pizza or in lentils, in apple pie or in tomato salad.

No matter what you have read in any previous diet, there is no special food that will slim you. The only way to slim is to reduce your calorie intake. And I'm going to show you how you can cut those calories down to the right level for *you* within *your* eating preferences. No drastic alterations in what you eat. I'm going to show how you can turn a 'fattening' diet – the kind you've been eating up until now – into a slimming diet, and a healthy one.

Here are some actual examples of high-calorie diets turned, quite easily, into low-calorie, healthy ones.

· EXAMPLE ONE ·

Susan, an averagely active eighteen-year-old, weighs 11 stone. At 5 ft 6 in tall, she is $1\frac{1}{2}$ stone overweight. Her weight gain began at school but has become worse in the last year since she started college and began living away from home.

'I won't eat anything for breakfast except toast. I always have lunch in the college cafeteria, where choice is limited, and in the evening I like a fast-food meal as I can't stand cooking. I've no real food favourites though – I'm easy to please as long as things are quick and easy.'

Here's what Susan ate in a typical day:

Breakfast

2 slices toast from a large loaf, liberally
   spread with butter and marmalade   350 calories

Mid-morning snack

3 chocolate-covered Hobnob biscuits   240 calories

Lunch

1 Scotch egg, serving of coleslaw and
   serving of baked beans   620 calories

Mid-afternoon snack

1 small packet peanuts (2 oz, 55 g)	280 calories

Teatime

1 7-in cheese and onion pizza	470 calories
Salad of cress, peppers, lettuce with salad cream	60 calories
1 apple	40 calories
1 glass red wine	85 calories

Late evening

1 large slice bread liberally spread with butter	150 calories

Throughout day

Five cups white coffee with sugar	250 calories
Total	2,545 calories

This total is probably around 300 calories a day more than Susan should be eating and accounts for her steady weight increase. With minor changes to her diet, and no hunger, she can reduce the total to around 1,600 a day for a good weekly weight loss. The new-look day's eating (right) also matches up well with nutrition guidelines (see Table 3, Chapter 2) as it gives 57·5 g protein, 945 mg calcium, 65·5 g fat (equivalent to just over 35 per cent of her day's energy intake), 21 g (minimum) fibre, 11·5 g+ iron, approx. 100 mg vitamin C, 8 g salt and sugar well within the 12 per cent limit. To reduce her fat intake to well within the 35 per cent limit, she could swop the crisps for a banana.

Breakfast

2 slices toast from a small loaf, lightly spread with butter and reduced-sugar marmalade	190 calories

Mid-morning snack

2 fingers chocolate-covered wafer	110 calories

Lunch

1 Scotch egg, serving of baked beans, tomato salad	440 calories

Mid-afternoon snack

1 packet lower-fat crisps (1 oz, 30 g)	120 calories

Teatime

1 7-in tomato and cheese pizza	435 calories
Salad with oil-free dressing	20 calories
1 apple	40 calories
1 glass red wine	85 calories

Late evening

1 small slice bread lightly spread with butter	100 calories

Throughout day

Five cups coffee with skimmed milk and sweeteners	100 calories
Total	1,640 calories

· EXAMPLE TWO ·

Mary, thirty-eight-year-old mother of two pre-teen children, has a part-time morning job. She's 5 ft 2 in tall and weighs 10½ stone. Before she had children she weighed 8½ stone. Lately she's been trying to diet, without success, by cutting out between-meal snacks. 'Also, although I'm not very hungry at breakfast time, I've been trying to eat a good breakfast to "set me up" for the day. Even so, I'm very hungry when I get home at lunchtime.'

Mary has to cook an evening meal for the family at 6 p.m. 'So I'm always hungry again by ten, but I make do with a milk drink before bed.'

Here's what Mary ate in a typical day:

Breakfast

Average bowlful (2½ oz, 70 g) muesli with ¼ pint (150 ml) milk	340 calories
1 medium slice toast with butter and honey	180 calories

Lunch

2-egg omelette cooked in butter with 6 oz (170 g) crinkle-cut chips and 4 oz (115 g) peas	790 calories
1 'thick and creamy' yoghurt and low-calorie squash	160 calories

Evening meal

Portion of a home-made cottage pie using traditional method	600 calories
4 oz (115 g) fresh carrots, boiled; gravy from powder	30 calories

Late evening

Hot chocolate drink with full cream milk
and sugar, 1 Digestive biscuit .... 255 calories

Total .... 2,355 calories

Mary has been gaining weight on this diet because, as she isn't very tall, she probably needs only 2,000 calories a day. Although Mary believes she is doing her best to diet, she is making several mistakes. There's no point in having a big breakfast if you don't really want one. Cutting out snacks doesn't work if you simply eat more calories at your normal meals. And she's wasting calories on lots of very high-fat items when lower-fat ones would do just as well. Muesli, by the way, is a deceptive food: it weighs heavily and even a small bowlful is high in calories.

Here's a new-look day which should result in easy weight loss for Mary.

Breakfast

2 Weetabix with $\frac{1}{4}$ pint (150 ml) semi-skimmed milk .... 186 calories

Mid-morning

1 medium slice bread with low-fat spread and honey (taken to work) .... 130 calories

Lunch

2-egg omelette cooked in non-stick pan with a little butter, 4 oz (115 g) thick-cut chips and 4 oz (115 g) peas .... 480 calories

19

Evening meal

Portion of a home-made cottage pie using Junk Food Diet method (see recipe, page 272)	300 calories
4 oz (115 g) fresh carrots, boiled; gravy from powder	30 calories

Suppertime snack

1 medium slice toast with low-fat spread and cheese spread	130 calories
1 slimmer's instant hot chocolate drink	40 calories
Total	1,296 calories

Mary's new diet is also sound nutritionally as she gets 66 g protein, 830 mg calcium, 39 g fat (equivalent to 25 per cent of her day's energy intake), 31 g fibre, 12 mg iron, approx. 58 mg vitamin C, approx. 7 g salt and sugar less than 7 per cent of total energy intake.

· EXAMPLE THREE ·

Twenty-three-year-old Jack works as a delivery man for a city furniture store. He is 5 ft 9 in tall, weighs 12 stone and would like to lose a stone. He shares a flat with other men. Living a typical bachelor existence, he snatches food when and where he can and has a takeaway most days. Evenings are often spent in the pub.

'I feel that my diet is unhealthy but I don't know what to do. I can't sit around eating cottage cheese and raw vegetables; my workmates and flatmates would laugh at me.'

Here's what Jack ate in a typical day:

Breakfast (7.30 a.m.)

2 Shredded Wheat with ⅓ pint (200 ml) milk .... 270 calories

Snack (10.30 a.m.)

Cheese and pickle sandwich from sandwich bar .... 350 calories approx.

Lunch (1.30 p.m.)

1 McDonald's Quarterpounder Cheeseburger .... 496 calories
1 large Cola .... 167 calories

Snack (4 p.m.)

Yorkie Bar .... 360 calories

Snack (7 p.m. – back at flat)

Ham and pickle sandwich .... 300 calories approx.

Drinks (8–10 p.m. – in pub playing darts)

3 pints beer .... 600 calories

Evening meal (10.15 p.m.)

Takeaway beef curry with rice .... 900 calories

Throughout day

Coffees with milk, no sugar	180 calories
Total	3,623 calories

A new-look day for Jack means he can still have several snacks and meals, and visit the pub, but the calories are greatly reduced. With a little fruit added, he now has a diet well within the COMA guidelines at 102 g protein, 65 g fat (28 per cent of day's energy total), 25 g fibre, 12 mg iron, 120 mg vitamin C, 900 mg calcium, salt at approx. 9 g and sugar level low.

Breakfast (7.30 a.m.)

2 Shredded Wheat with $\frac{1}{3}$ pint (200 ml) skimmed milk	220 calories
Small glass orange juice	40 calories

Snack (10.30 a.m.)

1 packet crisps (1 oz, 30 g)	140 calories

Lunch (1.30 p.m.)

1 McDonald's Quarterpounder (no cheese), diet Cola and 1 piece fresh fruit (taken to work)	444 calories

Snack (4 p.m.)

1 Crunchie bar	165 calories

Light meal (7 p.m. — bought from frozen counter on way home)

1 Birds Eye Captain's Pie (10 oz, 285 g)	
4 oz (115 g) frozen peas	345 calories

Drinks (8–10 p.m. — in pub)

3 half pints beer	300 calories

Evening meal (10.15 p.m.)

1 piece Tandoori chicken takeaway	280 calories

Throughout day

Milk for coffee (milk at home is skimmed, but whole milk used during day)	142 calories
Total	2,076 calories

So there you have the proof that it isn't difficult to cut down on calories while still eating plenty, and still eating the way you like! And, by following the Junk Food Diet, you'll do just that. It lets you eat all your favourite foods within a healthy, overall plan.

Here is a list of the many benefits of following the Junk Food Diet:

· It takes account of your own likes and dislikes. There's plenty of choice on the first part, the Set Diet. But when you begin the second part, the Pick Your Own Plan, there's almost unlimited flexibility.

· It's easy. There are no complicated menus, recipes or calculations. You can eat as simply as you like.

· It's familiar. There are no unusual dishes or exotic

ingredients to worry about. You'll find all the meals and snacks you know.

· It's convenient. You pick the way you want to eat. There are meals suitable for any situation, and there's a special 'Eating out' section.

· You won't go hungry. Before you begin dieting, we find the right calorie level for you, so you won't go hungry by following a diet that's too meagre.

· It doesn't make you enemies! Most diets don't get the approval of your family and friends. This one will, because family and friends will hardly notice you are dieting.

· It doesn't deprive you. You decide what foods you really can't live without, and the Junk Food Diet says yes, you *can* eat them!

· It's for life. When you've slimmed down to the size you want to be, I show you exactly what to do next so you don't put the weight back on – ever!

· A SUMMARY OF WHAT YOU'VE READ IN CHAPTER 1 ·

· There is no such thing as a 'junk' food or a 'health' food, only a good diet or a poor diet.

· A poor diet is a limited diet.

· A good diet is a varied one.

You *can* lose weight *and* eat healthily on a diet that includes all your favourite foods.

TABLE 1

TOP TEN FAVOURITE FOODS IN THE UK

Slimmers and non-slimmers alike

Women	Men
1 Bread	1 Meat
2 Chips	2 Chips
3 Chocolates/sweets	3 Chinese food
4 Meat	4 Curry
5 Spicy food	5 Bread
6 Potatoes	6 Potatoes
7 Chinese food	7 Pastry/pies
8 Cake	8 Chocolates/sweets
9 Fruit	9 Burgers
10 Fish	10 Fried fish

People actively trying to lose weight

1 Bread	6 Fruit
2 Chocolate/sweets	7 Cakes/biscuits
3 Poultry	8 Salad
4 Cheese	9 Takeaways
5 Meat	10 Fried foods

2 · HEALTHY EATING
THE FADS AND THE FACTS

Deaths from coronary heart disease (CHD) in the USA have been falling steadily every year since 1968; in fact, there has been a quite dramatic one-third reduction among men in the 45–64 age group.

'Ah!' says the health food lobby gleefully, 'a perfect example of how enlightened eating can help us beat our twentieth-century diseases!'

In fact, it isn't. For the first four years of CHD decline, fat consumption in the States actually *increased* to a record level of nearly 45 per cent of energy intake. And after twenty years that level is still around 40 per cent – much higher than the recommended level and as high as the fat consumption in the UK, where CHD has *not* shown a similar drop.

By mentioning these facts I don't infer that the advice the experts have given us to eat less fat is not valid. I simply point out that when it comes to the links between diet, health and disease, evidence and opinion are often contradictory. Out of all the speculation, debate, clinical research and field trials, very little proof of these links has actually been forthcoming.

Even the UK government's COMA report (see Table 2) agreed that all the evidence its panel reviewed 'fell short of proof', even though they felt it wise to give advice on the basis that the dietary measures recommended would certainly do us no harm and would probably do at least some good.

This kind of caution doesn't go down well with people

who desperately want to believe that we can cure or prevent all our ills by the food we eat – or the food we avoid. Health through diet is a very appealing concept as an alternative to our modern dependence on medicine and surgery. And it is a short step from *wanting* something to work, to *believing* it really does work and then to *crusading* for the cause. And that is how 'healthy eating' myths spring up. Unproven theories become absolute facts, facts become exaggerated – by word of mouth, in print, on TV – and suddenly eating is a dangerous pastime.

The post-war concept of food as not only necessary sustenance but also fun, enjoyment and harmless pleasure has been virtually crushed out of existence. The years of plenty must be replaced by years of prudence; if not, we will have to take full responsibility for the consequences (namely, our own ill health). Eating in the eighties is a stressful, guilt-ridden occupation.

And yet I'm sure that the experts responsible for the dietary advice reports of the eighties did not intend to have this effect. After all, guilt and stress can cause illness too!

In fact, they didn't say don't eat red meat. They didn't say don't eat dairy produce. There was no mention of banishing sugar from your life, or abandoning salt. Even more important, we are living longer, healthier lives than ever before in the history of mankind, so we can't be doing it *all* wrong.

Let's stop worrying for a minute and take a sensible look at what really does constitute a healthy diet.

Much of the advice we have received in the past decade revolves around what I call 'negative nutrition', it's telling us what *not* to eat. But the basis of healthy eating is, and always has been, 'positive nutrition' – making sure that we get all the nutrients we need for growth, health and repair. These are:

Protein

The body's 'building blocks' for healthy growth and maintenance of muscle, organs, tissue, the whole works. Found in animal and plant foods.

Carbohydrate

Sugars, starches and fibres. They give us the energy (calories) we need to stay alive, move and maintain body weight – the body's petrol. Found in plant foods and milk produce but not in meat or fish.

Fat

Another fuel, and also provides essential fatty acids. There are three main types of fat – saturated, monounsaturated and polyunsaturated – in animal and plant foods.

Vitamins

Needed in minute quantities to help our bodies work properly.

Minerals

Again, needed in small quantities for growth and repair and to help regulate body processes.

We also need water, the major constituent of our bodies without which we would quickly die.

Most of us feed ourselves and stay in good health without ever referring to a nutrition manual and I don't intend you to cut out this list and take it with you to the supermarket. But just to show you that there are many,

many nutrients which we need and couldn't do without in the foods that we may feel guilty about eating, look at Table 3.

TABLE 2

UK – Dietary Recommendations by the Committee on Medical Aspects of Food Policy (COMA) Report, 'Diet and Cardiovascular disease', DHSS 1984.

Fat Reduce consumption to 35 per cent of total energy intake.
Cholesterol No specific recommendations.
Sugar Intake of sugar should not be increased.*
Salt Intake should not increase further and consideration should be given to decreasing it.*
Fibre No specific recommendations.*
Body weight Obesity should be avoided.

* The UK NACNE report, published by the Health Education Council, gave more specific recommendations. They suggested a maximum sugar intake of 12 per cent energy, that long-term salt intake should fall by 3 g per person a day and that fibre intake should increase long-term to 30 g per person a day.

USA – Joint Committee of the US Department of Health and Human Services and Department of Agriculture, recommendations to the public.

1. Eat a variety of foods.
2. Maintain reasonable weight.
3. Avoid too much fat.
4. Eat foods with adequate starch and fibre.
5. Avoid too much sugar.
6. Avoid too much sodium (salt).

TABLE 3

WHAT OUR BODIES NEED FOR HEALTH*

Nutrient	What it does for you	Recommended daily amount	Best sources
Protein	Builds, repairs and replaces tissue	47–62 g (F) 60–84 g (M)	Dairy foods, meat, fish, poultry
Carbohydrates	Source of energy	Up to 55 per cent of total energy intake	Bread, potatoes, cereal, sugar
Fat	Source of energy and supply of transfatty acids	Up to 35 per cent of total energy intake 80 g (F) 110 g (M)	Oil, butter, lard
Fibre	For correct functioning of digestive system	25–30 g	Pulses, cereals, nuts, fruit, vegetables
Iron	Vital for oxygen transport around body	12 g (F) 10 g (M)	Red meat, offal, eggs
Calcium	For formation and maintenance of bones and teeth	500 mg	Dairy produce, fish, white bread, green vegetables
Vitamin A	For vision, skin	750 mg	Dairy produce, yellow and orange vegetables, offal, butter

TABLE 3 *continued*

Nutrient	What it does for you	Recommended daily amount	Best sources
Vitamin B1 (thiamin)	Helps convert food into energy	1 mg	Pork, rice, bread, potatoes, pulses
Vitamin B2 (riboflavin)	As above	1·3 mg (F) 1·6 mg (M)	Milk, meat, cereals, eggs
Vitamin B3 (niacin)	As above	15 mg (F) 18 mg (M)	Meat, offal, fish, cereals, beans
Vitamin B6 (pyridoxine)	Assists body functions	2 mg (F) 2·2 mg (M)	Meat, fish, eggs, poultry, potatoes
Vitamin B12	Helps form new cells	3 ug	Offal, meat, dairy produce. (No plant sources)
Folic Acid	As above	400 ug	Offal, green vegetables, pulses, cereals
Vitamin C (ascorbic acid)	For healthy tissue and healing	30 mg	Citrus and berry fruits, green vegetables
Vitamin D	For correct calcium utilization	10 ug	Oily fish, butter, margarine
Vitamin E (tocopherol)	Protects body fats	10 mg	Nuts, seeds, vegetable oils, eggs, cereal

TABLE 3 continued

Figures from the Ministry of Agriculture's *Manual of Nutrition* (HMSO) with the exception of the figures given for fibre (based on NACNE recommendations), fat (based on COMA recommendations), and vitamins B6, B12 and E and folic acid (all of which are the official USA recommended daily amounts).

F = female   M = male

* Recommended daily amounts given are for adult women and men in normal health. Babies, children, teenagers, pregnant and lactating women, the elderly, the ill and the convalescent require different amounts of certain nutrients. See Chapter 11 for advice for those up to eighteen years old.

So you can see that many of the foods we often worry about eating are the ones that are best at providing the nutrients we need for good health. And because the nutrients we need are so widely spread amongst the foods available to us, the crucial factor in good nutrition is to get variety into your diet.

On the Junk Food Diet, that important nutritional balancing act works very well indeed. Let's look at the foods and nutrients that have caused — and continue to cause — the most uproar in recent years, sort out the reality from the myths and see just how the Junk Food Diet copes with the official recommendations.

FAT

By the late seventies our fat consumption was over 40 per cent of our total energy intake. 35 per cent is the new level to aim for. The other thing we should try to do is eat less saturated fat (the kind found in animal and dairy produce) and more mono- and polyunsaturated fats (the kind found in plants).

Now, for anyone who wants to lose weight, to cut down on fat a little is sensible, as fat contains more calories (9 per g) than either carbohydrate or protein (both 4 per g). But cutting down *a little* is what we're talking about here. That 35 per cent goal — or a slimming target — in no way means that we have to give up our favourite meats, cheeses, milk and so on.

You could probably achieve the 35 per cent figure by doing nothing more than cutting visible fat off your meat before you eat it and using a low-fat dairy spread in your sandwiches instead of butter straight from the fridge (when fat is cool and hard, you can't spread it thin). On the Junk Food Diet you will cut down your fat intake to well within acceptable levels because we're reducing the overall calorie content of your diet and, therefore, the fat content.

Before we leave the subject of fat, here's a novel piece of advice that you're not likely to have read anywhere recently: I don't think it is a particularly good idea to reduce the amount of fat in your diet to much below the official recommendations in the belief that if less is good, virtually none must be even better. In particular, I don't think you should give up red meat. I say that for the following reasons:

• Foods which contain animal fat are also excellent sources of some of those vital nutrients we looked at in Table 3. Red meat is second only to offal as the best source of easily absorbed iron (it is three times as easily absorbed into our bodies as the iron found in plant foods). Give up red meat and you'll have to work quite hard, especially if you're female, to get enough iron in your diet – chicken and fish contain very little. Red meat is also an important source of vitamin B12, and this is why vegans, who eat neither meat nor dairy produce, have to be careful not to go short of this vitamin.

• Lean beef, pork and lamb all contain a high proportion of protein.

• Contrary to what people think, the fat in red meat isn't all the saturated kind. Far from it. Mono- and polyunsaturated fat account for over two-thirds of the fat in meat. And if you choose your red meat wisely, you are not getting a very high-fat food in any case.

Neither does it appear advisable to try to raise the amount of polyunsaturated fat (such as seed oils) that you eat either. Major trials have shown that while these fats lower blood cholesterol levels, thus reducing the risk of CHD, they probably increase the risk from other diseases. Much more research needs to be done, but meanwhile – take it easy!

· SUGAR ·

Long before fat became public enemy number one, sugar was the nutritional baddie. There were two main reasons.

First, it is the only food that contains no nutrients apart from energy. Nothing but calories! And at 112 calories per 1 oz (30 g), it is quite high in those calories too.

Second, the evidence incriminating sugar as a major cause of tooth decay is strong.

Now it also appears that there is a link between high sugar consumption, mid-life-onset diabetes and heart disease: certain studies have found that people who consume high levels of sugar are more prone to both diseases.

You may also have heard that sugar is physically addictive, a kind of drug. It is true that sweet foods are the ones most likely to tempt you to eat when you aren't hungry (how many desserts have you succumbed to after claiming you were full up?). It is also true that if you eat a high sugar sweet or snack when you are hungry rather than a more balanced meal or snack, the sugar sets off a chain reaction in your body that has the end result of lowering your blood sugar levels – and helping you to feel you need more sugar. However, this doesn't add up to addiction, and despite the near catalogue of complaints against sugar, I still believe that you *can* enjoy a certain amount of sweet food – even if you're slimming – without feeling guilty.

The Junk Food Diet's message is that sugar is no big deal – if you want some, you can have it, but in a sensible way. I've made sure you get all the nutrients you need for good health within a certain calorie level, and *then* I've put a fairly generous calorie allowance on top for whatever sugary items you fancy. I also give guidelines on how and when to eat sweet foods, for the sake of your teeth as well as your health. (If you *don't* have a sweet tooth, we use those calories for other treats instead.)

· SALT ·

Although it is quite true that most of us eat a lot more salt than the 3 g per day our bodies actually need (in average circumstances) for good health, it is not true to say that salt is a direct cause of high blood pressure or that a drastic reduction in consumption would result in any particular health benefits for the majority of us. All that has been proved is that if you do suffer from high blood pressure (hypertension) and you cut your salt intake, your blood pressure may be lowered.

It is estimated that one in five of the population will be at risk from hypertension, and lowering salt intake would be a good idea for those people. (A visit to your doctor to clarify your degree of risk and have a blood pressure reading will help you and your doctor decide whether you are one of those who would benefit from a low-salt diet.) For the remaining 80 per cent of us, it should be more than adequate to cut our consumption by 3 g or so a day, as NACNE recommended. If, as most of us probably do, you have been eating around 12 g a day, that represents a 25 per cent cut, which, in fact, is not difficult to achieve. Let's look at the sources of the salt in our daily diets. One-third occurs naturally in our food: for example, in meat, fish, in vegetables and even in fruit. One-third is added during food processing not only to foods that taste salty, such as smoked bacon and corned beef, but also to a wide variety of other foods, such as breakfast cereals, tinned soups, tinned spaghetti, pickles, tomato ketchup and bread. One-third is the salt we add ourselves, in cooking and at the table.

On the Junk Food Diet it is easy to cut your salt intake, if you want to, by simply not adding salt to your meals at the table, and by gradually reducing the amount you add to your cooking. It is easy to cut down even more, if you like, by choosing lower-salt or no-salt items in the supermarket. And more about that in Chapter 4.

If you don't like the sound of cutting down a little on your salt, all I can tell you is that I did exactly that after twenty-five years of eating a lot of salt – and within only two days I found the small reductions I was making completely acceptable.

· FIBRE ·

The fibre mania reached such a level of lunacy a year or two ago that I began to wonder whether the food manufacturers were going to start adding bran to cheese, fish fingers and choc ices in a bid to increase sales. Fibre was the nutritional hit of the decade.

Now the excitement has died down a little (even to the extent that white bread sales are on the increase again), the population falls into two camps – those of us who stick with our wholegrain cereals and our pulses and swear by fibre as a cure for almost everything, and those of us who adore white spaghetti and patna rice and would do almost anything to avoid eating a prune.

If we fall into the latter category, are we doing ourselves untold harm? Probably not.

It is a fact that if we suffer from constipation and we then increase the amount of fibre-rich foods in our diet, the constipation will almost always be cured. A fibre-rich diet is also useful in preventing or minimizing associated problems such as irritable bowel, diverticulitis (when swellings develop in the walls of the large intestine – a disease common in people over fifty) and haemorrhoids (piles), said to affect up to 10 per cent of the population. But all the other cases for fibre are still the subject of debate.

If you are in normal health without the above problems, it could be that you are already getting plenty of fibre in your diet, and increasing it won't achieve anything. People's fibre needs do vary a great deal, and the 30 g per day that NACNE recommend may actually be too much for many of us.

Few of us will actually need more than 30 g a day: and very high intakes of bran may impede your body's ability to absorb calcium, iron and zinc, all three essential minerals. So again, don't think that if some is good, more must be better.

In any case, you don't have to eat lentils and brown rice every day in order to get good amounts of fibre. Although it doesn't occur in animal products, only in plants, there is fibre in all kinds of food – yes, even white spaghetti and polished rice! You can eat plenty of 'junk' food and still get all the fibre you need, fibre that will help you to slim because it will help you to feel full and satisfied. Look down the list in Table 4 and you're bound to find some foods that you like. On the Junk Food Diet, you pick and choose your fibre foods to suit yourself. The Set Diets contain on average 25 g of fibre per day, with extra optional.

TABLE 4

FIBRE IN YOUR FAVOURITE FOODS

	Fibre (grams)
Baked beans, 8 oz (225 g)	16
Processed peas, 5 oz (140 g)	11
Frozen peas, 4 oz (115 g)	9
Raspberries, 1 bowful	8·5
Chilli con carne, average serving	7
Dried apricots, 'no need to soak', 1 oz (30g)	6·5
Pease pudding, average serving	6·5
Canned garden peas, 5 oz (140 g)	6
Wholewheat pasta, average serving	5·5
Baked potato, 1 × 8 oz (225 g)	5
Shredded Wheat, 2	5
Stoned dates, dried, 2 oz (55 g)	5
Weetabix, 2	4·8
Baked apple	4·5
Instant mashed potato, average serving	4·5
Shelled almonds, 1 oz (30 g)	4
Banana	3·5
Carrots, 4 oz (115 g)	3·5
French beans, 4 oz (115 g)	3·5
Crisps, small packet	3·5
Avocado, $\frac{1}{2}$ medium	3
Grapenuts, $1\frac{1}{2}$ oz (45 g)	3
Medium slice Hi-Bran bread, 1 oz (30 g)	3
Mushrooms, 4 oz (115 g)	3
Medium slice wholemeal bread, 1 oz (30 g)	2·5
Nectarine	2·5
Orange	2·5
Strawberries, average serving	2·5
Dessert apple	2

Digestive biscuits, 3	2
Medium slice granary bread, 1 oz (30 g)	2
Popcorn, 1 oz (30 g)	2
Sultanas, 1 oz (30 g)	2
White pasta, average serving	2
Sugar Puffs, 1 oz (30 g)	1·7
Melon, average slice	1·5
Peach	1·5
White rice, average serving	1·5
Cornflakes, 1 oz (30 g)	1
Medium slice white bread, 1 oz (30 g)	1
Peanut butter for 1 slice bread	1

· CALCIUM ·

Calcium is the latest nutrient to come under the spotlight. Its role in minimizing or preventing osteoporosis, a debilitating weakening of the bones which affects one in four women over sixty-five and one in forty men, has been the subject of much media attention, but once again, there is no absolute agreement amongst the experts about exactly how big a role calcium plays, nor about exactly how much calcium we should be getting in our diets.

The UK Department of Health recommended daily amount is 500 mg for adults; in the USA the figure is 800 mg, and the UK National Osteoporosis Society recommends up to 1,500 mg per day.

One fact is certain: an adequate calcium intake is essential to make, and keep, strong bones. The denser your bones, the less trouble osteoporosis should cause in old age. And on the Junk Food Diet, your richest source of calcium – dairy foods – isn't limited drastically. Neither does the diet frown on white bread, which, unlike wholemeal bread, has calcium added.

TABLE 5

VITAMIN C IN FAMILIAR FOODS

	mg
Blackcurrants, 4 oz (115 g)	200
Orange	70
Strawberries, 4 oz (115 g)	70
Kiwifruit	60
Melon, average slice	50
Orange juice, 4 fl oz (120 ml)	40
Small can tomatoes, 7 oz (200 g)	35
Sweet potato, 4 oz (115 g)	25
Instant mashed potato, 4 oz (115 g)	20
Pineapple rings, 2	20
Chips, 4 oz (115 g)	15*
Courgette	15
Peas, frozen, 4 oz (115 g)	15
Roast potatoes, 2	12
Nectarine	10
Tomato	10
Sweetcorn, frozen, 4 oz (115 g)	7
Canned peaches, average serving	4

*Depending upon the age of the potatoes, preparation and cooking method and other variables, content can be much less.

· VITAMINS ·

On a varied diet, even a low-calorie one, you're unlikely to go short of vitamins. Every food you eat, apart from white sugar, contains something that's good for you!

Perhaps the hardest vitamin to get enough of is vitamin C. A regular supply is vital as your body doesn't store it, and apart from a little in liver and milk, vitamin C is found only in fruit and vegetables.

Junk food lovers often have an aversion to vegetables, especially to cabbage and other 'greens'. But if you're a greens-hater, you can still get plenty of vitamin C: how about peas, or potatoes – even chips are a good source – or sweetcorn, or tomatoes?

If you're not keen on any vegetables at all, try fruit: soft fruits, peaches, nectarines, melons and all citrus fruits are great sources of vitamin C. Don't like fruit either? How about fruit juice?

And don't forget, your fruit and vegetables don't have to be fresh: frozen and canned both contain vitamin C too. On the Junk Food Diet I'll make sure you get your vitamin C one way or another!

· FOOD PROCESSING ·

Processed food was frequently mentioned in my survey (see Chapter 1) as a prime example of what was meant by 'junk food'. And yet processed foods make up nearly three-quarters of the British diet! If this figure sounds high, it is simply because a large proportion of food in its 'natural' state isn't fit to eat. Processing, for instance, turns cereal grains into bread and breakfast cereals. It also makes available to us a gigantic variety of foods that would otherwise be unavailable – out of season vegetables can be frozen and out of season fruits canned, for instance.

It is true that there are some highly processed products on sale that are low on nutrients and high on that other scapegoat of the eighties – additives. Long-shelf-life cakes, pies and pastries are probably as near to genuine junk as you will find – and yet even so, a slice of 'eat within two years' fake-cream sponge cake or a pack or two of instant pudding mix now and then aren't going to harm you. Food additive intolerance appears to be yet another area for doubt. A recent large trial involving 10 per cent of the entire population of a large UK town resulted in only three people showing 'clinically definable' intolerance.

Despite trial results such as these, food additives are a very sensitive area, and this is why the food manufacturers are busy removing more and more additives from their products. In fact, they are doing their best to ensure that the quality of canned and convenience foods is higher than ever before.

You could eat a perfectly healthy diet without ever having to go near a fresh food again. Table 6 gives an example of a day's healthy eating without any fresh foods in it at all. (Chapter 4 deals in more detail with processed foods and your diet; Chapter 11 deals specifically with children and food processing.)

TABLE 6

A DAY'S HEALTHY EATING* INCLUDING NO FRESH FOODS

Breakfast

2 Weetabix with $\frac{1}{2}$ pint (150 ml) long-life semi-skimmed milk
4 fl oz (120 ml) long-life orange juice
1 crispbread with 2 teaspoons honey

Lunch

3·5 oz (100 g) can tuna in oil, drained
5 oz (140 g) canned potato salad
3 oz (85 g) portion vanilla ice cream
$\frac{1}{4}$ can apricot halves in juice or syrup, drained
1 large glass lemon squash

Snack

2 oz (55 g) sultanas

Evening meal

4 oz (115 g) beefburger (frozen), well fried
5 oz (140 g) instant mashed potato
6 oz (170 g) mixed carrots and peas, canned
Individual carton long-life custard 5½ oz (150 g)

Snack

1 packet salted crisps

Throughout day

⅓ pint (200 ml) semi-skimmed long-life milk in tea and coffee

*For an 8½-stone adult woman on a maintenance diet.

This day's diet provides: 1,850 calories (some women may need more than this to maintain their body weight); a low fat content of just over 30 per cent of the total energy intake (62·6 g, 563 calories); 27·3 g fibre; 18 per cent of total energy intake in protein; 52 per cent energy intake in carbohydrates; 89 g vitamin C; 876 mg calcium; 13·43 mg iron; 1,468 ug vitamin A; 1·32 mg vitamin B1; 2·81 mg vitamin B2; 32 mg vitamin B3; 1·81 mg vitamin B6; and 8 ug vitamin B12. Total added sugar content of the diet is 56·4 g, or 12 per cent of total energy intake.

Healthy junk indeed!

· TAKEAWAYS ·

Finally, the remaining great subject of debate amongst

students of healthy eating – are fast food takeaways poor nutritional value, and how often should you eat them?

All takeaways fit into one of three categories:

> many good points and few, or no, bad ones;
> some good points and some bad ones;
> many bad points and few good ones.

No takeaway meal on earth can be described as 100 per cent junk. But how to sort out the excellent takeaway from the poor one? I've devised a checklist of good points to look out for, with the corresponding bad points.

GOOD	BAD
Very recently prepared/cooked	Been prepared/kept warm a long time
If fried, fresh, clean, unsaturated oil used at correct temperature	Fried in animal fat/over-used oil at too low a temperature
Contains at least 10 per cent protein	Contains very little protein
Contains reasonable amount of fibre	Contains little fibre
Contains not more than 35 per cent fat	High in fat
Contains vitamin C	No vitamin C
High nutrition to calories ratio	Low nutrition to calories ratio
Low to average salt content	High salt content

Scoring 1 for every good point and 1 for every bad, let's look at a few popular takeaways.

Beefburger in white bun with relish, from national burger chain

Scores 5 good points and 2 bad (lowish in fibre and contains no vitamin C). Second category doesn't apply. So, on balance, a beefburger is a good takeaway. (If you eat a lot of takeaways, it's always wise to get them from national chains because turnover is high and certain standards always apply: for example, food is prepared and cooked when your order is placed whenever possible and standard ingredients, portion sizes and cooking methods are usual.)

Doner kebab

Scores 8 good points and no bad ones – excellent takeaway!

Pizza from national chain

Depending upon the variety you choose, pizza scores from 4 to 8 good points and 0 to 4 bad ones. Some pizzas contain more fibre and vitamin C than others and some are quite high in fat and/or salt, largely depending on the amount and type of cheese in them.

Fish and chips from local shop

Fish and chips varies enormously in its nutritional value from shop to shop. A portion of white fish in batter with chips from a 'greasy chip shop' with low turnover may give you a very high calorie, high saturated fat, low vitamin C meal with hardly any fish (therefore hardly any protein) inside the batter. Bad point score could rate up to 6! On the other hand, a standardized, well-cooked portion of fish in a *thin* coating of batter and chips from a chain could yield all good points and no bad ones.

Chinese and Indian takeaways are the hardest of all to categorize because there is no standardization. But in general you can use common sense to get a reasonably good estimate of good and bad scores. If a beef curry is swimming in visible fat, for instance, it is safe to assume it is high in fat altogether.

So is it sensible to indulge in takeaways or not? Yes, I think it is! They are by no means the nutritional baddies they are often made out to be. Not by a long way. But of course, no one can force you to buy a balanced meal: beefburger, milkshake and apple pie, for instance, may well put your day's diet in total disarray, whereas beefburger, orange juice and French fries might have been the perfect meal!

· TAKEAWAY TIPS ·

· Choose a popular busy national chain where you're likely to get the best nutritional value.

· Takeaways that include no freshly cooked chips or potato and no fruit or fruit juice, vegetables or salad will contain no vitamin C. Add a piece of fresh fruit yourself, or make sure you get C-rich foods at another time in the day.

· Don't think of a takeaway just as a small snack in between main meals; think of it as a meal in itself.

· Use common sense when choosing a complete takeaway meal. Get some carbohydrate (bun, rice, bread, chips) plus some protein (meat, fish, cheese, egg) and no more than one high-fat item (pastry, chips, thick batter) and you can't go far wrong.

So there you have virtually all the good news about your diet. But here's some news that may cheer you up even more, as you are about to embark on your diet to shed that unwanted weight.

If you slim you'll be doing your health the biggest favour of all.

In the fight against chronic illness and complaints of many kinds – including heart disease – a slim body is your greatest ally. Being overweight can cause or aggravate all the following conditions; being slim will help you to avoid them, minimize them – or even cure some of them them:

· Heart disease, high blood pressure and strokes.
· Mid-life-onset diabetes.
· Bronchitis, asthma and other respiratory disorders.
· Arthritis and other joint disorders.
· Varicose veins, piles, gallstones and hernia.

In addition, increasing degrees of obesity in men are statistically linked with increased risk of colon, rectum and prostate cancers. Increasing degrees of obesity in women are statistically linked with increased risk of breast, uterus and cervical cancer.

The fact is that it is being overweight and not specific dietary components which is the biggest threat to our twentieth-century Western health. In other words, it's not so much *what* you eat as *how much*.

Do yourself a favour and lose that weight.

· A SUMMARY OF WHAT YOU'VE READ IN CHAPTER 2 ·

· Healthy eating does not mean you have to give up fat, sugar and salt and all your favourite foods.

- Healthy eating is as much about getting enough of all the nutrients you need as it is about cutting down on others.

- Fat-containing foods can be a useful part of your diet.

- You can enjoy a certain amount of sugar in your diet without feeling guilty.

- Salt may not be a health hazard for most people, but it's easy to cut down the salt in your diet if you are an 'at risk' person.

- Some of us are worrying needlessly about getting a lot of fibre in our diets.

- You can live quite healthily on a diet of processed foods.

- By no means all takeaways are poor food.

- One of the best ways to help your health is to lose weight.

3 · EATING TO SLIM
MYTH AND REALITY

If you had lost an ounce for every ludicrous dieting 'fact' that I have read, been told or overheard during the past decade, you wouldn't need to lose weight now, that's for certain.

So much nonsense is talked and written about the subject of dieting that it is amazing people can keep finding new things to make up. Yet find them they do. And that is why I want to take some time here to 'clear the decks' and clear your head of all those half-remembered 'truths' and half-forgotten myths so that you won't be sidetracked or ambushed when you begin slimming this time.

Let's look at how you are most likely to have come by ridiculous dieting advice.

· SLIMMING FOLKLORE ·

One of the earliest dieting 'facts' was first announced around twenty years ago when, so we were told, a grapefruit eaten before every meal would help you slim because it 'burnt up' the calories in your food. Remember?

Well, surprise, surprise; just when we all thought the grapefruit theory had been consigned to the dieting dustbin, it had a revival, this time in the form of grapefruit pills, marketed a couple of years ago most successfully – presumably because all of us old enough to have been around the first time had forgotten that they didn't work.

I think dieting myths are a bit like a favourite pair of worn-out slippers: we know they're useless but we don't want to throw them out. Foods that are supposed to 'burn up' other foods or the fat in your own body are top of the league. I know people who swear that protein, eaten in the form of a steak or a chicken leg, for example, 'burns off' your fat, and that that is why a high-protein diet slims you down. But only if you eat the protein with *no* carbohydrate, folks! (So what happens if you eat protein plus grapefruit – a carbohydrate – I wonder?) Talking of high-protein diets, I also often hear that these work because the body can't convert excess protein into fat. (It can, and it does, if you aren't getting enough calories from the carbohydrate foods.)

You've probably got some more folklore of your own. Well, now you know what to do with it.

· 'SCIENTIFIC' THEORIES ·

'Nutritional breakthrough!' 'Amazing new diet theory!' 'Scientifically tested way to slim!'

I have hundreds of diet books on my office shelves that promise slimmers the earth and quote pseudo-scientific tests and theories. Over the past decade or more, various authors have told us, as if it were proven fact rather than mere theory, that, for example, our bodies burn up calories better if we eat nothing except fruit until lunchtime. We have been told that the only way to get slim is to eat what we like, but in a certain order, so that the different types of food don't mix. We've been urged to take supplements of amino acids to alter our metabolic rates. And we've been assured that by taking large doses of certain vitamins we will also raise our metabolic rates.

Need I tell you that all these theories are, at best, unproven and at worst absolute rubbish. You may well lose weight by following a diet which heralds itself with pages of scientific-sounding mumbo-jumbo. But you will lose weight because the diet is low in calories, not because its author has made the one amazing breakthrough your digestive system has been waiting for all these years!

The famous Beverly Hills diet, for instance, sold us the barmy idea of 'combining' foods in certain orders and eating masses of 'enzyme-producing' pineapples and the like. But the diet actually worked to get the pounds falling off you fast because it was very, very low in calories.

So don't be fobbed off with an important-sounding diet which will have you scurrying around looking for out-of-season fruits or expensive pill supplements. You don't need them.

· 'BUT YOU MUST ...' ·

The sort of advice you are likely to get from friends – who are probably only trying to be helpful and encouraging – most frequently takes the form of things you 'must' and 'mustn't' eat when you're slimming.

They will be horrified if they see you tucking into a bag of crisps or enjoying a glass of wine. They will creep guiltily off to the vending machine and hide conspicuously behind the filing cabinet when they want to eat a bar of chocolate, never dreaming that you can actually *eat one yourself* if you want to.

The fact is that there are no hard and fast rules about what you must and mustn't eat on a weight-loss diet – only, I repeat, that you should take in fewer calories over the course of a day, or a week, than your body needs to maintain its current weight.

It's worth taking a closer look at the most-often uttered 'musts' and 'mustn'ts'; the kind of prejudices you'll be up against from everyone – including the family doctor, if you should ever happen to ask for advice on weight loss from that quarter. Not one of them stands up to close examination.

Read on – carefully – so you'll know *exactly* what to say in answer to the people who will be trying (in a well-meaning way, of course!) to make your life a misery while you slim.

'You must eat lots of salad when you're slimming'

Just why salad has got its reputation as obligatory food for people wishing to lose weight I'm not sure. True, lettuce, cucumber, tomatoes, cress and so on are very low in calories, but apart from that distinction, your traditional salad has little to recommend it. It will provide some vitamin C and some fibre, but it is by no means the best source of either, or of any other nutrient. It doesn't fill you up and it is so boring that many dieters, driven to distraction by their compulsory salad with their steak or their ham or their cheese, fall foul of what I call the Mayonnaise Syndrome. They dollop on great spoonfuls of dressing – be it mayonnaise, salad cream, French dressing or blue cheese dressing. Ah! That tastes better! But whichever dressing you choose, you can be sure of one thing – you just turned your goodie-goodie salad of around 25 calories into a 150-calories-plus plateful. The irony is that you could have had all the mashed potato you wanted, say, or two slices of bread instead.

If you don't like salad – don't feel obliged to eat it. Nothing dreadful will happen to you if you don't. I promise!

'You must eat more fish and poultry'

Steamed or grilled white fish is probably second only to lettuce in sending any would-be dieter off on a chocolate binge. If you're not a fish lover, apply the same philosophy. If you force yourself to eat it, you'll only end up breaking your diet. And if you do eat it, you're likely to pile on the tartare sauce or make up for your deprivation with a larger-than-average helping of French fries.

Yes, fish is a good source of protein, and even if you can't face more than the occasional coley or plaice fillet, you may find you like trout or rich and meaty monkfish, for instance. But by no means all fish is as low in calories as cuts such as cod, plaice and haddock are, at around 22 calories per oz each. Salmon and sardines are around 50 per oz, herring is 65 and so is mackerel. So don't be fooled into thinking that all fish is lower in calories than meat. It isn't.

Very lean beef (a lean cut, reasonably well roasted or grilled and trimmed of visible fat) is only 40 calories per oz. Lean mince, cooked then drained of fat, is the same. So you see, there's nothing to say you shouldn't eat red meat on your diet. And with butchers paying more and more attention to giving us less fat meat all the time, you shouldn't feel guilty about eating a burger or a steak instead of a piece of fish or chicken. Chicken meat, by the way, is 40 calories per oz without its skin. With its skin, it goes up to 60 – proving nothing except you should eat chicken only because you like it and not because someone told you it's less fattening than red meat!

'You must eat a good breakfast when you're dieting'

According to a survey by the Consumers' Association, only 75 per cent of the population in the UK eat breakfast every day.

If you happen to be one of the 25 per cent who doesn't and then you are told by some bully-boy of a diet that you must, first, you will feel resentful, and second, you will, more than likely, put weight on.

Some people (and I am one of them) are genuinely not hungry when they first get up. It seems silly, then, if you are trying to cut back on the amount you eat, to stuff several hundred calories down yourself at a time when you could gladly do without them. Much better to save the calories for a snack later in the day when you do feel hungry.

So why do so many people, nutritionists and slimming club leaders included, say you *should* eat a 'good breakfast'? If you're slimming, the theory is that if you miss breakfast, you will undoubtedly feel starving by mid-morning and binge then.

It is also claimed that you will feel faint and lack concentration throughout the morning if you don't eat breakfast. Well, I feel all right, but only you know how you feel, and whether or not eating something before 9 a.m. helps you feel any better. Probably, if you always eat breakfast and feel hungry at that time of day, then you would suffer if you gave it up. If you're a non-breakfast eater, then for heaven's sake, don't start now!

'You must re-educate your palate to diet successfully'

In certain cases 're-educating' your palate can be helpful. For example, it takes only a fair degree of willpower over a three-week period to change from being a dyed-in-the-wool user of three spoonfuls of sugar in your tea to someone who pulls a face if she detects as much as a few grains of sugar in the cup. Similarly, when you reduce the amount of salt you use in cooking and at the table, it is amazing how quickly your previous 'normal' amount tastes quite foul. So, helping your taste buds to get used to less sweet tastes, for instance, can be very useful.

But no amount of 'palate conditioning' will work to help you slim unless you re-educate your mind first! You've got to want to lose weight and you've got to be convinced that you *can* do it – more about that in Chapter 5.

'You mustn't eat fried food on a diet'

There's no mustn't and no must about it, but you *can* if you want to.

Although on the Junk Food Diet you will be reducing the overall fat content of what you eat, that isn't to say you can't eat some fat, and some of that fat can be in the form of fried foods if that is what you really like.

Some fried foods aren't as fattening as people will have you believe. Take fried eggs. One average raw egg is about 80 calories. Fried in hot oil and well drained on a slotted spoon before being served, it will contain only about 120 calories. That's 40 calories' worth of fat, or around 4·5 g – less than a teaspoonful of oil.

By cooking foods quickly in very hot oil you can save a lot of calories. Put frozen chips into oil that isn't hot enough and they'll sit around soaking up the fat until they start cooking. They will be twice as high in calories as thick-cut chips cooked for a little time in really hot fat. And frying big items rather than small ones can save you hundreds of calories – forget whitebait and go for a big chunk of cod!

Shallow frying certain foods can actually be no more fattening then grilling them. For instance, if you start bacon off in a warm, non-stick pan brushed with oil and gradually heat it up until its own fat starts to run out, then you turn the heat up and fry until the bacon is golden and crisp, and then you drain the bacon well when you serve it, it will have no more calories than if you had grilled it. This also applies to sausages (well cooked), steak and burgers. When fatty meat cooks, by whatever means, it loses fat; it doesn't absorb it.

Lastly, stir-frying is a great way to fry if you're watching calories. You don't have to have a wok; a non-stick pan will do. Add a couple of teaspoons of oil, your favourite thinly sliced meat and vegetables, and, if you keep stirring while you cook over a high heat, adding perhaps a little stock or soya sauce along the way, you have a dish that smells, looks and tastes wickedly high in calories but isn't at all.

'You mustn't snack between meals'

Not true. Not only is snacking between meals not harmful to your diet; it could be an advantage!

First, to know that you can have something to eat other than at breakfast, lunch and dinner (or tea), is very comforting when you're dieting. It stops you from feeling deprived. If you aren't 'allowed' to snack, you are much more likely to cheat and eat that chocolate bar anyway.

The anti-snackers say that between-meals snacks will

make you fat because you eat them as extras to your ordinary meals. But of course that doesn't have to be the case at all. The Junk Food Diet will show you how to include snacks within your day's slimming diet!

Second, several small meals a day help to keep your metabolism working at top efficiency; in other words, you may get slim a little quicker by eating, say, five snacks rather than two big meals a day.

So if you enjoy snack eating, don't try to change!

'You mustn't eat starchy foods when you're slimming'

I can hardly believe it when I hear it, but I still get slimmers telling me proudly that they are on a high-protein diet and being 'good' by cutting out bread and potatoes.

So if someone is plugging that idea to you as the best way to slim, ignore them. The 'starch' foods like rice, pasta, bread and potatoes are a valuable part, both practically and nutritionally, of your slimming diet.

Potatoes cooked plainly have only 25 calories or less per oz, compared with 120 for a 'protein' food like Cheddar cheese. Cooked rice and pasta have 35 per oz and bread has 60 to 70. So it's the 'stodge' foods that help fill you up when you are on a diet, as well as providing vital nutrients, without giving you too many calories. They are the backbone of any decent diet that isn't going to leave you ravenously hungry, and, as you will find out, on the Junk Food Diet I don't believe in you being ravenous at all.

'You mustn't drink alcohol on a diet'

There are certain people who shouldn't drink alcohol whether or not they are dieting: for example, if you are under medical orders not to do so, if you are taking certain prescription tablets, if you are pregnant or if you are trying to conceive.

Otherwise, if a glass of wine with your evening meal, a pint of beer after work or a Scotch when you get home is your idea of a treat, then I see no reason at all why you shouldn't continue to enjoy it on a slimming diet.

Alcoholic drinks aren't all that high in calories: a glass of wine is about 90 calories, a single measure of spirit is 50 and half a pint of ordinary beer is 90.

On the Junk Food Diet, your daily treats allowance can be taken in alcohol, if you like, without you feeling guilty, because I have made sure that the limit is within the government's guidelines for good health. I will also show you how to cope with those special occasions, like your birthday, when one glass or two just doesn't seem enough!

Of course, if you have been a habitual ten pints a night man, then that could explain why you need to lose some weight, and you are going to have to make some compromises here.

Certainly, if you've been used to having more than a couple of drinks a day on a regular basis, then I would suggest cutting down, not only to help you lose weight but also for your health's sake. I managed to more than halve my own consumption of my favourite tipple, white wine, by mixing it, at first half and half, and then a third to two-thirds, with sparkling mineral water. I now find I actually prefer the watered-down version!

Here are some more tips to help you control the amount you drink:

- Drink your fill of water before you start on alcohol so that you're not thirsty;
- Sip don't gulp;
- Put your glass down between sips;

· Try alcohol-free wine or beer.

Heavy drinking comes down to habit in most cases, just as overeating does, so if you can find easy ways to break the habit, the rest is simple.

If none of my tips works, or if you can't even bring yourself to try them, consider getting professional help.

'You mustn't eat cakes, biscuits and puddings on a diet'

It is true that you could blow a whole day's calorie allowance on a couple of items if you chose unwisely: for instance, 1,000 calories would be gone in a flash if you decided to eat one good slice of cheesecake and a big helping of Black Forest Gateau with cream.

On the other hand, you could have a slice of sponge, a couple of sweet biscuits *and* a chocolate mousse and still have enough calories left over to have a nutritious day's eating on 1,000 calories a day.

A little of what you fancy *does* do you good, so don't try to diet by cutting out all the things you like best. It just won't work.

'You mustn't touch chocolate – one taste will end in a binge'

Not if you are on the Junk Food Diet, it won't!

I know that many people think of chocolate as a demon to be banished from their lives before it overtakes them completely, but it *can* be bullied into shape and take its place legitimately in your diet.

The secret is to allow for it within your slimming campaign, enjoy it, savour it, eat it – and don't feel guilty. Then get on with your life and your diet.

What *does* end in a binge – be it a binge of chocolate or sweets, bread or oatmeal cookies – is a long spell of deprivation.

You know the scene. You start a diet, one of the many that limits your choice of food, especially of the one food you really like. You stick to the diet for a few days, even a week or two. You're proud of your strong willpower and your few pounds of weight loss. You've said 'No' to your favourite food, you've won the battle!

Then, half-way through day three, or day seven, or day ten, for no reason that you can really explain, you surrender. You walk into the kitchen quite intent upon grabbing a crispbread and an apple, and somehow you walk out with a handful of chocolate-coated biscuits. Or you pop into the corner shop for a magazine on your way home from work, and without even knowing *you* did it, you buy two Mars Bars (maybe three). They are all gone by the time you get home. And then, feeling a failure, you will sit down and polish off a plate of jam sandwiches.

You won a battle but you lost the war. 'What does it matter anymore?' you say. 'That's one more diet down the drain. I just *can't* diet. I haven't got the willpower.' And it's a long, long time before you think about losing weight again.

Yet it's not your willpower at fault, it's the diet, for making you exercise superhuman willpower in the first place. The deprivation method of dieting can't work for most of us for more than a few days.

For more about how you can eat chocolate – and all the other 'binge' foods – while you slim, and for more about how you can stop thinking of a diet as a battle-ground where temptation will always beat you, turn to Chapter 5.

· A SUMMARY OF WHAT YOU'VE READ IN CHAPTER 3 ·

· Think very carefully before accepting advice you read or hear about slimming: it's probably wrong!

· There are no hard and fast rules about what you must or mustn't eat on a diet: as long as you reduce your overall food consumption, you will lose weight.

· It is not true that you must eat salad, lots of fish and poultry, a good breakfast, regular meals or a great deal of high-fibre food in order to lose weight.

· It is not true that you mustn't eat fried foods, starch foods, between-meal snacks, cakes, puddings, biscuits or chocolate, or drink alcohol while you're dieting.

· The only successful way to slim is to include your favourite foods in the diet.

4 · SUPERMARKETS
USER-FRIENDLY SHOPPING

Have you ever wondered why the people you see going in and out of health food stores don't appear to be any more healthy than the rest of us?

There is certainly no proof that people who avoid supermarkets live longer and healthier lives than the 75 per cent of us who happily drive that giant trolley once a week.

And I'm not surprised. I believe that supermarket shopping is by far the best bet for anyone who wants their diet to be nutritious, slimming and tasty. And here are my reasons why:

· Virtually everything that can be bought at a health food store (with the possible exception of a handful of specialist vegetarian or vegan processed items) can be bought at the supermarket chains, but the opposite is far from true, even when it comes to 'healthy' items. For instance, where a health food store may offer one or at most two varieties of muesli, the supermarket will offer five or more. There is far more choice of *everything*.

· The supermarkets have a high turnover of produce so you can be sure of fresh foods. Quality is also closely monitored and standards are high.

· Fresh fruit and vegetables are kept in perfect conditions. Having been packed and transported correctly, they are then displayed for sale in cool conditions, often with specially dimmed lighting, which helps preserve maximum vitamin content. Most health food stores (and, come to that, market traders and corner shops) don't have the knowledge, the facilities or the room to do this, and produce kept in warm, light (sunlight is worst of all) conditions, and perhaps kept for a week or more when trade is slow, will lose up to 100 per cent of its vitamin C – a vitamin vital to your good health. A good-quality supermarket tomato is worth twenty organically grown but badly stored health shop tomatoes.

• Supermarkets have a wide range of foods suitable for slimmers, most of which are calorie-counted. Portions are standardized and controlled and low-calorie alternatives to high-calorie foods are always stocked. Health food shops, on the other hand, carry little calorie information or special slimmer's products (apart from, ironically, expensive courses of 'slimming pills', which *won't* be on your Junk Food Diet shopping list anyway).

• Most supermarkets even provide calorie information on the 'naughty' foods like pre-packed cakes and pastry products, so you can easily build them into your diet. And if you want even more information, on fat or sugar content, for instance, that's provided on many foods too.

• Most supermarkets have additional nutritional information available for you: full calorie-counted lists of products, diet booklets, family meal planners, healthy eating leaflets, recipe leaflets and so on.

In addition to all those plus-points, prices on comparable items are almost always lower at supermarkets, with the possible exception of some items sold 'loose' such as shelled nuts, herbs and spices. So stop feeling guilty every time you pass the health store by. Instead, I'm going to take you now on a special slimmer's guided tour of the much-maligned supermarkets to show you exactly how much they can help you on your diet. But first, to avoid or get round the few pitfalls you will come across as you shop, take note of these tips:

· Take a list. Casual, unplanned, haphazard shopping (whether it's for food or clothes) always results in you getting home with things you didn't want, things you already have more than enough of, and things you wish you could take straight back. If it's clothes you probably *will* take it back; if it's food, you'll probably eat it.

· Don't ever shop when you're hungry. It is amazing how much more sweet or stodgy foods you think you need when you wheel your trolley round the aisles just before lunchtime, faint from starvation. Don't do it. Eat your food, then do your shopping. You'll save £££s as well as lbs.

· If you haven't many items on your list, use a basket not a trolley.

· Get tough about special offers. Even armed with your list, it is tempting to buy six six-packs of jam tarts just because they are a few pence cheaper this week — even if you don't like jam tarts! Only buy things you like or need, things you have room for in the larder/fridge/freezer, and things that won't spoil or rot before you have time to eat them.

Now let's get on with that tour . . .

The chilled dairy cabinets

Here you'll find a splendid array from the most fattening to the least fattening foods you can buy! Slimmers can certainly forget the far-off days when the choice was natural cottage cheese or nothing. The manufacturers have done wonders in producing all kinds of lower-calorie cheeses, and the best news of all are the reduced-fat versions of our favourites, such as Brie, Cheddar, Edam, Cheshire and cheese spreads. Calorie savings range from 25 per cent to 50 per cent, which will always be explained on the pack. As well as supermarket own brands, look out for Shape, Delight and Tendale reduced-calorie cheeses.

Full-fat cream cheese has 125 calories per oz. I find the skimmed milk soft cheese, which is supposed to be an acceptable substitute, tastes and looks like school chalk. But the *half fat* soft cheeses are very nice – and only 50 calories per oz. Even the dreaded cottage cheese can be quite nice these days: it comes in dozens of varieties and some brands are very creamy.

More and more of us are turning to skimmed milk and away from full-cream (whole) milk. But if you are one of those people who still find the taste of skimmed milk too thin, it is worth trying semi-skimmed. You still save 115 calories a pint and, if no one tells you, I swear you'll never know the difference! If you use dried milk powder, don't forget that many have added fat. Only a few (such as Marvel) don't. Read the label carefully.

Moving on to the fats section, you'll see that butter takes up much less space than it did a decade ago and in its place are all kinds of 'spreadables'. Some of these, but by no means all of them, contain only half the calories of butter. All these will be clearly labelled 'low-fat spread'. Some brand names to look out for are Gold, Delight, Outline and Clover Light. Although I still use – and love – butter for cooking and as a garnish, I always use a low-fat spread now for sandwiches. Again, I defy anyone to tell the difference if they haven't been told beforehand! And they spread so easily and so thinly you save even more calories that way too – butter straight from the fridge doesn't so much spread as go on in chunks.

If you're wondering whether to buy oil instead of butter

for cooking, to save calories, oil (all kinds) actually has more calories than butter. At 250 calories per oz it's the highest-calorie food in the world! Buy corn or sunflower oil rather than blended vegetable oil if you're watching polyunsaturates.

The meat counter

Whether you buy your meat fresh or frozen, there's no difference nutritionally and all the advice that follows applies to either.

If you're slimming, there is no need to pass the red meat counter by. Beef, pork, bacon and lamb can all be lower in calories than chicken or turkey! This is for two reasons. First, the meat producers are bowing to popular request and producing cows, pigs and sheep with a higher lean to fat ratio. In other words, there is less fat in traditional cuts of meat than there was a decade or so ago. Second, many butchers now prepare the various cuts of meat in the Continental style, which means there is less waste and less visible fat. Of course, many butchers still stick to their old methods, but the leading supermarkets are one step ahead in the race to give us leaner meat. While they still offer fattier cuts, you will always find a selection of leaner cuts too. These will be marked either 'less than 10 per cent fat' or 'lean choice', and you should find mince, stewing meat, braising meat, fillets, steaks and cutlets to choose from. These cuts are a bit dearer but there's absolutely no waste so the cost is no higher in real terms.

If you don't find any meat marked 'low in fat', simply have a good look at the cuts available and pick one which seems to have least visible fat. Everyone thinks pork and lamb are fatty, but their lean meat is no more fattening than chicken at 40 calories per oz. So the message when buying meat is avoid the fatty cuts. Belly cuts, breast and shoulder of lamb are amongst the fattiest there is! Duck, by the way, isn't too bad if it's *well* cooked. Most of that fat will have melted away into the pan.

If you like bacon and sausages for breakfast, you'll notice that, like the red meats, they come in extra lean versions too. Low-fat sausages have an extra high lean meat content and some bacons are labelled 'lean choice'. However, if you can't find these, don't worry too much — ordinary sausages become low-fat sausages when they're well grilled and you can easily trim most of the surplus band of fat off bacon rashers before cooking them.

The frozen cabinets

These are full of good things for slimmers. Dozens of ready meals, almost all calorie-counted, and most are quite low in calories too. There's so much variety, with recipes from all over the world, that dieting really becomes fun. They are ideal for cheats — in order to get second helpings you have to buy two packs!

Other frozen foods ideal for dieters are individual pizzas or pizza slices, French bread pizzas, individual pies, stir-fries, all the various crispy-coated fish and poultry fillets and goujons, and burgers, all of which can be baked, microwaved or grilled rather than deep fried.

Sweet toothers can choose ice cream as a reasonable low-calorie dessert, but beware the family-sized frozen puddings and gateaux unless you really do have a hungry family. Once defrosted, you can't cut off just one small slice, can you?

Frozen fruits and vegetables are perfect slimmer's fare. If you live alone, you can pour just what you need, so there's no temptation to 'finish up the can'. And the vitamin C content of frozen fruit and vegetables is high. If you are fed up with chips, you can try the dozens of other potato products to grill, ovenbake or microwave.

Canned produce

Even if you have a freezer, you may want to stock up on some canned meats, fish, fruit and vegetables – in fact, anything you can get fresh, you can get in a can. If you are one of those people who equate cans with 'nasty additives', it's worth thinking again. Canning is a method of preservation in itself, so the addition of further preservatives and anti-oxidants is unnecessary. The quality of canned food largely depends on the quality of the food when it was fresh. And canning *doesn't* destroy all the vitamin C in fruit and vegetables.

Depending on the product, the can may have added sugar or salt. But if you look hard along the shelves you will probably find low-sugar baked beans, spaghetti and fruits, all of which will save you some calories. And if you're watching your salt intake, you'll find low-salt alternatives too.

(There are surprisingly few E numbers in canned produce, but for more on that subject, read on to the end of this chapter.)

Jars

Down in the preserves aisle you can find low-calorie versions of almost all your favourites. There's low-sugar jam and marmalade and reduced-oil mayonnaise and salad cream, all of them saving 50 per cent of the calories. There's oil-free French dressing for almost no calories a spoonful as opposed to 120, and tangy seafood sauce with a 50 per cent saving. Or how about low-calorie tomato ketchup and low-fat meat pastes and spreads?

Packets

Don't forget a pack of instant mash, some dried fruit and nuts for nibbles, some rice and pasta for quick meals and plenty of cereals for breakfast. You can also find sprinkle sweetener to use instead of sugar on your cornflakes, or pill sweeteners for your morning coffee. Artificial sweeteners have come a long way since straight saccharin; the new generation are hard to tell from sugar. That's why all those calorie-free squashes and canned fizzy drinks are so nice now – talking of which, you could put some of those in your trolley too.

· THE ADDITIVES QUESTION ·

Should you feel that you are doing your body untold harm if you buy packs, jars or cans of food with E numbers in them?

A major recent controlled British trial sponsored by the Ministry of Agriculture has shown that allergic reaction to additives – indeed, to any foods, including natural ones such as wheat – is much rarer than we have been led to believe. If you know that you are allergic to a certain food or additive, then of course you should avoid that food or additive. But 999 people out of 1,000 can eat foods containing E numbers and can both feel, and be, perfectly well and healthy. All additives in food on sale in this country for humans have been approved by the government after extensive tests and so the blanket idea that all additives are in some way harmful for all people is one you can safely leave behind. Some additives, such as vitamin C and beta-carotene, can even be beneficial.

Having said that, the food manufacturers, ever eager to please the customer, have been exceedingly busy over the past few years removing all kinds of additives from their products. Nowadays it's quite hard to walk down an aisle in the supermarket and find a packet *without* the words 'no artificial colours', 'no artificial flavouring' or 'no artificial preservatives' on it. So the question of additives is gradually being taken out of our hands. But ironically, in its place, the question that food manufacturers are beginning to worry about is how they can make the public realize that foods without preservatives just don't last as long as foods with preservatives. Food poisoning from bacteria and moulds will no doubt be the hot problem of the next decade. If you choose foods without preservatives, you *must* remember to store them carefully according to the instructions on the packet and eat them within the 'best before' date, which is likely to be very soon, which leads me on to . . .

· THE FOOD POISONING QUESTION ·

A few straightforward precautions and tips can remove most of the risk from bacteria that currently appears to be involved in eating many everyday foods – including eggs, poultry, pre-cooked chilled meals and salads.

· Unless you're sure your source of eggs is salmonella-free, cook them thoroughly and avoid raw eggs, and runny poached, fried or boiled eggs.
· Cook all meat – especially poultry – thoroughly, and wash your hands after handling raw meats.
· Choose frozen ready meals rather than pre-cooked, chilled ones and follow cooking instructions carefully.

Never eat a ready meal which is not well cooked right through.

· Avoid unpasteurized soft cheeses – processed ones such as Philadelphia are fine.

· Re-wash salad stuffs when you get them home.

· Get your shopping home as soon as you can, preferably using an insulated bag for frozen and chilled products.

· Store raw and cooked foods separately.

· Make sure your fridge (5 °C max) and your freezer (−18 °C max) are at the correct temperature.

· Don't keep cooked food for more than two days.

· Remember those most at risk from food poisoning are babies under one, pregnant women, the ill and the elderly.

· A SUMMARY OF WHAT YOU'VE READ IN CHAPTER 4 ·

· You can buy all you need for a balanced, healthy diet at your favourite supermarket.

· When you shop, take a list with you.

· Don't be afraid to try all the reduced-fat items: cheeses, spreads, milk, lean choice meats, dressings and so on.

· Also try the reduced-sugar items like baked beans, jams and marmalades.

· Frozen ready meals are ideal for lone slimmers.

· Cans and jars are good stand-bys, and not bad for your health. Try low-calorie sauces, soups and canned puddings.

· 999 people out of 1,000 will come to no harm eating foods containing additives.

5 · SLIMMING SENSE

Anyone can lose weight on the Junk Food Diet – safely, permanently and healthily. It's the simple, perfect diet for most people.

But before you even begin to read the diet itself, and most certainly before you begin to diet, it is important – no, it's crucial – to get yourself into the right frame of mind for losing weight. Okay, you may *think* you're already in the right frame of mind ('I bought the book, didn't I?' 'Yes, but how many others did you buy and abandon straight away?') Spend a little time here with me now thinking about *you* and what you can *do* to guarantee slimming success at last. You may not find that all of what follows will apply to you, but some of it will. And you have my assurance that I haven't dashed off some tips in an idle ten minutes at the end of a busy day. This little bit of slimming sense is the result of ten years' experience and observation of all kinds of people on all kinds of diets. I've been fortunate enough to have had more opportunity than any nutritionist or doctor or psychologist to study the main reasons why people fail to lose weight, even given an excellent diet, and I've had plenty of time to work out solutions, many of them tested on myself, my family and friends!

· ARE YOU FRIGHTENED OF DIETING? ·

I know of hundreds of women for whom the mere sound of the

word 'diet' is enough to produce an instant nervous headache and a sudden need for the complete contents of the cake tin. Anyone who has witnessed a friend or colleague struggling through day two of their sixth diet this year consisting of lettuce and cottage cheese could, let's face it, be forgiven for having diet phobia and preferring to remain over-weight.

So many people equate dieting with deprivation, hunger, misery and a host of other negatives, is it any wonder that lots of us are secretly terrified of even contemplating a diet, however badly we need and long to lose weight?

Yet, until you can conquer that fear, you'll never be able to start a diet in the right frame of mind, let alone stick to one for more than a few days.

So let's look at the reasons for your fear.

Deprivation

Remember my promise to you – you don't have to give up the foods you like best on the Junk Food Diet. You don't have to eat foods you don't like. No Spartan regimes. No oddball ideas. So – no deprivation, right? Right.

Hunger

No. You will feel no genuine hunger on the Junk Food Diet. (I say 'genuine' hunger deliberately, because many, many people who have spent months or years or all their lives eating more than they need, confuse hunger with all kinds of other feelings. There will be more on that subject later in this chapter, and more detailed help in Chapter 10.) Genuine hunger is kept at bay because we pick you a dieting level that is right for your body, and that way you won't starve, or come anywhere near starving.

Fear of change

Diets often mean quite major changes in large chunks of our daily lives. After all, shopping, cooking, eating, drinking and 'food socializing' are a big part of most of our lives and, especially if we lack confidence in ourselves, we enjoy familiar routines associated with food. On the Junk Food Diet I have deliberately kept any changes you will have to make to an absolute minimum. But there is another kind of change that might, secretly, frighten you. You may not even realize you're a victim of it until you read the next few paragraphs. That change is the change in yourself if the diet is a success.

The more weight you lose, the more changes you will have to accommodate. Most of these changes will be the ones you long for – to be able to wear more fashionable clothes or a swimsuit on the beach, or to be healthier, for instance. Everyone who loses weight agrees that the benefits are well worth the effort. But many people who aren't successful at slimming are frightened – perhaps subconsciously – of the effects these changes may have on their lives. If, for example, you've spent years being everyone's 'fat friend', a shoulder to cry on, you may worry that you'll lose your identity, that you'll no longer be needed. Or perhaps you've become used to being the unattractive one, always ignored by the opposite sex. How will it feel if you suddenly become desirable? Or if you married your husband or wife when you were overweight, what will being slim do to your marriage? Will you be tempted by affairs? Will he/she get jealous of your new looks? Will your friends get jealous? And so on . . .

There aren't any easy answers to these doubts and fears, but if some strike a chord with you, we've probably hit upon the exact reason why you haven't lost weight up until now. You're not so much frightened of dieting, you're frightened of being slim, of being someone unfamiliar!

Which is why I'm going to tell you now that being slim may make you look better, feel better and increase your self-confidence, but it won't turn you into someone completely different. People who genuinely love or like you now will still love or like you when you are slim. If you lose a 'friendship' through changing your body shape, was that 'friendship' really solid or worth hanging on to by staying fat? Equally, if you married your partner only because he or she was the one person who wanted you when you were fat, you may find you want to look round again when you're slim. But if you genuinely love your partner, you'll still be together when you've lost weight.

Fear of upsetting other people

I'm always amazed at the number of potential slimmers who don't start a diet because they are frightened of upsetting family or friends – not by the long-term results of the diet, but by short-term inconveniences. And it is quite astounding how selfish other people can be when it comes to your diet! If money rates as the biggest cause of marital rows, then I'm sure that diets come second. And if you have tried to cope with a diet and the tantrums and sulks that go with it, no wonder you're worried about starting another one!

So why do other people tend to react so unfavourably to your diet? All sorts of reasons. Maybe your bad temper while on previous diets has caused it. Maybe you're a diet bore, talking endlessly about calories and ounces lost. Perhaps you make everyone else feel guilty for not being on a diet, or you force everyone else to eat 'rabbit food' too (husbands, especially, are in dread of this). Lastly, both friends and lovers hate the wet blanket effect that a diet often has on your social life. You won't go out for a meal or to the pub — or if you do, you sit there sipping slimmer's tonics.

Well, you can forget *all* of that hassle on the Junk Food Diet. You needn't even bother to tell friends and family that you're dieting. They'll never find out, except by looking at your shrinking poundage, of course!

Fear of failure

If you have been an habitual dieter, starting dozens but never getting beyond day two of any, you'll know only too well the guilt, and perhaps the shame, of failure. And the more often you've failed to lose weight, the more inevitable it becomes with each new dieting attempt.

Even if you *say*, 'This time I'm really going to do it', underneath you're thinking, 'Why should this time be any different? In fact, why even try? Why not just admit that I'm meant to be fat and tell everyone I'm happy as I am? Or why don't I buy the diet book and say it didn't work because I have a slow metabolism?'

If fear of failure is your reason for not even trying any more, look at it this way. Which is worse: trying one more time (but *really* trying this time) or being overweight, needlessly and guiltily, for the rest of your life?

I devised the Junk Food Diet for confirmed dieting failures. It doesn't induce fear, it beats it. There are no punishments for not losing a certain amount of weight in a certain time, or for a few mistakes along the way. So go for it — you, yes even you, *can* do it!

· WHAT'S YOUR HURRY? ·

What every slimmer really wants is to lose weight *and never put it back on again*. The most successful way of doing that is to slim slowly. The least successful way – by a mile – is to crash diet.

So *why* are you in so much of a hurry to lose weight? Whether you've half a stone to lose or five stone, losing weight too quickly is going to *waste* your time, not save it! Here's why.

If you haven't much weight to lose

The temptation is to follow the quickest crash diet you can find so you can get the diet out of the way and start eating normally again.

So you find your very low-calorie diet, stick it out for a week, lose your weight and feel very pleased with yourself. 'I can't be bothered messing about with slow diets,' you tell your friends smugly, and you go back to your pre-crash normal diet. Within two days (yes, only two days) you've put back 3 lb. And within another two weeks, you've put back all of the weight you lost. Now you'll have to do it all over again – if and when you can be bothered to muster up the willpower to get through another week or so of deprivation. And I've got some very bad news for you. Next time, it's going to be harder. There is evidence to show that people who continually lose weight, then put it back on again, also gradually replace their lean muscle tissue with more and more fat, so that each time you diet, although you may get down to your target weight, the muscle that gives your body its nice shape is getting less and you're getting flabbier and flabbier! And that nasty flab fat is harder to shift than that original fat was the first time you dieted.

What is more, there is evidence to show that repeated diets have the cunning effect of lowering your body's metabolic rate, with the result that at the end of every new diet, you can't eat as much as you used to without putting on weight again. Literally, the more you crash diet, the less you can eat without getting fat! Horrible thought!

If you have a lot of weight to lose

Crash dieting will give you a slightly different set of problems. First, though you may be able to stick a very Spartan diet for a week, can you really stick it week after week after week? If you can, you're the exception. Most people will give up and feel a failure. Then, of course, most very low-calorie diets won't be giving you enough of all the nutrients you need, so you could be putting your health at risk with deficiencies. You could even be threatening your life by shedding lean muscle tissue (including tissue from vital organs such as your heart) instead of fat.

Lastly, and probably most importantly, if you have a little or a lot to lose and you do succeed in crashing it off, you're missing the most vital role of a good diet: to help you learn how to eat in the future so that you don't put the weight back on. So please, don't be in a hurry!

· DO YOU BELIEVE IN MIRACLES? ·

If you're still patiently waiting for that wonderful slimming miracle to come along, the one where you eat whatever you like but still lose weight, you're not ever going to succeed on a down-to-earth, calorie-controlled diet.

It's so tempting to put your faith into an expensive magic

diet pill or a cream that melts the fat away. Then, when it doesn't work at least there's the consolation that it wasn't your fault you didn't lose weight. But in the long run, where does that get you? Certainly not any slimmer. So, for anyone who is still always tempted by advertisements claiming dieting miracles of one kind or another, here is my definitive list of lotions, potions and slimming 'aids' that just *do not work*.

- All pills that claim to slim you while you continue to eat what you like. This includes 'starchblockers', said to stop all starchy foods being absorbed by your body.
- 'Slimming creams' that you rub into your skin.
- Suits that you wear to 'melt the fat away'. All these suits do is help you sweat off a pint or two of liquid when you exercise. The increase in calories burnt up when you wear one is minuscule.
- Laxative pills, which have no effect at all on the surplus fat that is already in your body and an adverse effect on your digestive system if taken more than occasionally.

True, you can go to your GP or a private doctor or slimming clinic, ask for, and perhaps get, one of several slimming pills on prescription which may well help you to lose weight (if you can put up with the unpleasant side-effects and the possibility that you will become dependent on them), but then you have the same old problem – you come off the pills and back comes the weight, which is the main reason I am totally against prescription pills.

So if you can't believe in miracles, what can you believe in?

Well, how about yourself? Believe in yourself and your own ability to be in full control of your own life, including your eating habits. First, think of yourself as a slim person. Think of being the size and shape you want to be. Think of buying clothes in the size you want to be and *can* be. Imagine yourself with the confidence to apply for a new job because your appearance is so much better than it used to be. (Don't let the feminists convince you otherwise: overweight people *are* discriminated against in the job market.)

This will all help you to stop seeing yourself as a fat person. So many overweight people tell themselves, 'This is just the way I'm meant to be.' The longer you've been overweight, the more inclined you are to accept the way you look as right for you. So get out of that way of thinking. Be positive and determined that you will slim. And don't let anyone tell you otherwise. I know many a would-be dieter who has stayed fat and 'happy' for years, thanks to friends or family who insist upon saying things like, 'Oh, you're lovely as you are. You're just big-boned. We're not a family of skinnies. Your face will go all gaunt if you lose weight.' (You can probably think of some more.)

Of course, if you say for the twentieth time this year, 'I'm going on a diet', no one will believe you. So if this *is* your twentieth diet, perhaps this time you would be wise to not mention it. Just get on and do it, and wait for everyone to say, 'Oh, you've lost weight. Don't you look wonderful!'

I explained earlier in this chapter why some people may do anything they can to stop you slimming. So please *don't* believe them when they say you were meant to be fat. You were not. Just believe in yourself.

· *WHEN FOOD IS THE ENEMY* ·

Many overweight people eat too much because food is their friend, a crutch to be turned to in times of worry, stress, boredom or misery. Then suddenly, when they try to diet, not only has that crutch been taken away but food has become the enemy. Suddenly, every day seems to be one long battle.

Now, how about this for a change in thinking. Enjoy your food! Enjoy tastes and textures and aromas. Accept food for what it is — enjoyable and necessary fuel for your body, the means of keeping you alive, healthy, fit and strong. But it is not the mystical holder of special powers over you, not a substitute for friends, love, sex, hobbies, work or anything else.

Get food back into perspective, stop battling, start relaxing and enjoying it, and then, and only then, will you become a successful slimmer and an ex-fattie for life. On the Junk Food Diet you can eat any food that you want to eat, so there is no need, ever, to crave cake or freshly baked bread and feel that you aren't allowed it. Therefore there's no need to eat the whole cake or the whole loaf, because it's always there. It's not going to run away.

· HELPING YOUR DIET ALONG ·

Having got yourself in a positive frame of mind for your diet, there is still more you can do to ensure success.

Don't waste calories

Never eat a high-calorie food or drink a high-calorie drink when a low-calorie one would do just as well. For instance, if you don't mind low-fat spread on your sandwiches, then don't waste calories on butter. If you can take sweeteners in your coffee instead of sugar, then have them. Saving calories whenever you can means that you will have some to spare for the foods you really like.

Choose the right time to begin your diet

If you're in the middle of moving house, getting divorced, giving up smoking, taking exams or have just got the sack, this may not be the perfect time to start your diet. You are probably too preoccupied to give it your best.

Choose a time when there are no major upheavals or disappointments in your life. And a special note for women: just before your monthly period may not be a good time to begin a diet either, as many women retain fluid and/or feel stressed at this time of the month; wait till day five.

Get motivated

If you have some specific as well as general reasons for losing weight, you may find it helps a great deal.

For instance, although it may well be enough for you to want to be healthier or to fit into smaller clothes, how much better to aim for one or two specific things: slimming for a holiday or a wedding. Or you could even buy an outfit that catches your eye and slim into it.

But one word of warning: if you use a specific date as your motivation, don't say something like, 'By my birthday I will lose two stone' (or whatever your ultimate target is). Simply say, 'By my birthday I will lose some weight.' You see, once you tell yourself you are going to lose a definite amount, if by any chance you fall short of that amount by the specified date, you will feel a failure and probably give up, which wasn't the point of the exercise at all! And so never, ever set yourself strict goals, let alone impossible ones.

· WORKING OUT HOW MUCH
WEIGHT YOU WANT TO LOSE ·

Knowing approximately how much weight you need to lose gives you something concrete to aim for. So although you don't have a target date, you do have a target weight.

If you don't know what you should be, here are some ways of telling:

If you have ever been at your 'normal' weight as an adult, what did you weigh then? You could aim for that weight again. (It's not true that you have to put on weight as you get older.)

Check the height/weight chart (Table 7). Half a stone or more above or below the average weight listed could be right for you. If in doubt, set your target at half a stone over the acceptable average listed. When you get there, you can always revise your target down a bit if you still look overweight.

What do you do if you want to lose weight and yet the height/weight chart says that you are well within the right weight for your height? Get the opinion of a sensible, unbiased friend or, failing that, a doctor or slimming club adviser. If the consensus of opinion is that you don't need to slim, it could be that you simply need to do some regular exercises to tone up your body. A non-existent waist, a protruding stomach and flabby thighs are three areas that all respond well to a short daily toning routine that will help you look slimmer even though you weigh the same. Which brings me on to the last point.

· SHOULD YOU EXERCISE? ·

If you've been an inactive person up to now, I think you should start building a little exercise into your day-to-day life as you lose weight. That way you burn off a few calories and you begin to realize that you have a body there that was made to do a bit of work now and then!

By exercise, though, I don't mean you have to or, indeed should, take up anything really strenuous such as jogging, weight training or squash. I was thinking more of a little daily walking.

And then I think you should try to do some body toning exercises at least three times a week while you diet. That will help any loose skin to shrink back to size and will help give you the sleek, slim look that dieting alone never quite manages to achieve, unless you are very young or very lucky. Ten to fifteen minutes is all you need, concentrating on your 'worst' areas – any reputable exercise book or video will help you, but don't choose an advanced programme until you are advanced.

Now, all the talk is over and it's time to lose some weight!

· A SUMMARY OF WHAT YOU'VE READ IN CHAPTER 5 ·

· Most people have some mental block that stops them from slimming. Find yours for success.

· Don't be in too much of a hurry to lose weight: the only way to slim and never put the weight back on is to slim slowly.

· Believe in yourself, not in dieting miracles.

· Food isn't your best friend or your deadly enemy. Learn to relax around it.

· Help your diet to help you.

· Take a little exercise.

TABLE 7

HEIGHT/WEIGHT CHART FOR WOMEN*

Height	Average weight	Acceptable weight range
4 ft 11 in	104 lb	94–122 lb
1·5 m	47·25 kg	42·75–55·5 kg
5 ft	107 lb	96–125 lb
1·53 m	48·75 kg	44–57 kg
5 ft 1 in	110 lb	99–128 lb
1.55 m	50 kg	45–58 kg
5 ft 2 in	113 lb	102–131 lb
1·58 m	51·5 kg	46·5–59·5 kg
5 ft 3 in	116 lb	105–134 lb
1·60 m	52·75 kg	47·75–61 kg
5 ft 4 in	120 lb	108–138 lb
1·63 m	54·5 kg	49–62·75 kg
5 ft 5 in	123 lb	111–142 lb
1·65 m	56 kg	50·5–64·5 kg
5 ft 6 in	128 lb	114–146 lb
1·68 m	58 kg	52–66 kg
5 ft 7 in	132 lb	118–150 lb
1·71 m	60 kg	54–68 kg
5 ft 8 in	136 lb	122–154 lb
1·73 m	61 kg	55·5–70 kg
5 ft 9 in	140 lb	126–158 lb
1·76 m	63·5 kg	57–72 kg
5 ft 10 in	144 lb	130–163 lb
1·78 m	65·5 kg	59–74 kg
5ft 11 in	148 lb	134–168 lb
1·81 m	67 kg	61–76 kg

* Weight without clothes.

HEIGHT/WEIGHT CHART FOR MEN*

Height	Average weight	Acceptable weight range
5 ft 4 in 1·63 m	130 lb 59 kg	118–148 lb 53·5–67 kg
5 ft 5 in 1·65 m	133 lb 60·5 kg	121–152 lb 55–69 kg
5 ft 6 in 1·68 m	136 lb 62 kg	124–156 lb 56·5–71 kg
5 ft 7 in 1·71 m	140 lb 63·5 kg	128–161 lb 58–73 kg
5 ft 8 in 1·73 m	145 lb 66 kg	132–166 lb 60–75·5 kg
5 ft 9 in 1·76 m	149 lb 68 kg	136–170 lb 62–77 kg
5 ft 10 in 1·78 m	153 lb 69·5 kg	140–174 lb 63·5–79 kg
5 ft 11 in 1·82 m	158 lb 72 kg	144–179 lb 65·5–81 kg
6 ft 1·83 m	162 lb 73·5 kg	148–184 lb 67–84 kg
6 ft 1 in 1·86 m	166 lb 75·5 kg	152–189 lb 69–86 kg
6 ft 2 in 1·88 m	171 lb 78 kg	156–194 lb 71–88 kg
6 ft 3 in 1·91 m	176 lb 80 kg	160–199 lb 73–90 kg
6 ft 4 in 1·93 m	181 lb 82 kg	164–204 lb 75–93 kg

* Weight without clothes.

6 · THE JUNK FOOD DIET – 1
PICK THE PLAN FOR YOU!

The Junk Food Diet begins right here! And the first thing we must do is ensure that you'll be eating the right amount for *you* on it – an essential that many diets forget.

An active girl of twenty-one, for instance, will need many more calories a day when she's slimming than a fifty-year-old inactive woman, even if they both want to lose the same amount of weight. And, conversely, two thirty-year-old men of the same height will probably have different calorie requirements depending on how much they want to lose and what exercise they take. That's why, with the help of my special slimmer's questionnaire below, we find the perfect plan for you. And that's why *anyone* can lose weight on the Junk Food Diet.

The diet itself, no matter how many calories a day you are on, is in two stages. First there's a Set Diet, lasting a minimum of two weeks. You'll start on between 1,000 and 1,500 calories a day, depending upon your answers to the questionnaire. Then, if you have more weight to lose, you either stay on your Set Diet or, if you prefer, you move to the Pick Your Own Plan, an ultra-flexible diet that allows you maximum control over what you eat, when you eat, how you eat and where you eat. I have simply taken all the hard work out of dieting for you on this plan (as you'll discover in Chapter 8) until you're right down to target weight.

· FINDING YOUR CALORIE LEVEL ·

Below are eight crucial questions with a different score for each answer. All you have to do is pick one answer to each question and write the appropriate score in the box at the end of the line. When you've answered all the questions, add up your score and check what it means. (Do be honest with yourself about the answers to questions 5–8, because bending the truth will only result in you getting the wrong score, and perhaps the wrong diet!)

The questionnaire

	Available score	*Your score*
1. Your sex:		
Male	5	
Female	1	1
2. Your age:		
21 or under	4	3
22–30	3	
31–50	2	
51 or over	1	
3. Your height:		
Over 5 ft 11 in	4	
5 ft 6½ in–5 ft 11 in	3	8
5 ft 2½ in–5 ft 6 in	2	
5 ft 2 in or under	1	
4. Amount of weight you need to lose:*		
Over 3 st	5	13
2 st 1 lb–3 st	3	

89

1 st 1 lb–2 st	2	
1 st or less	1	

* See page 84 in Chapter 5 if you need help on this

5. **Your working/regular day is:**

Very physically active – spend most of time on the move (e.g. sports teacher, builder)   3   ☐

Fairly physically active – spend several hours a day on feet (e.g. sales assistant, postman)   2   ☐

Sedentary – spends less than one hour a day on the move (e.g. word processor operator, receptionist)   1   14

6. **Amount of exercise taken (over and above that covered by question 5):**

Regular – at least three times a week – sustained – at least thirty minutes a time – aerobic activity (e.g. jogging, swimming, cycling)   3   17

Regular sustained mild aerobic activity (e.g. walking)   2   ☐

Little or no regular sustained exercise   1   ☐

7. **Dieting history – choose whichever of the following statements is closest to your experience:**

Haven't dieted at all in recent years   3   20

Often start diets, lose a little, give up, never get down to target   2   ☐

Have got down to target at least once, but always put it back on again   1   ☐

Have been losing weight recently on
another diet   1   ☐

8. **Choose whichever of the following
statements most closely matches your
ideal diet:**
I prefer to lose weight very slowly if it
means I can eat a little more   3   ☐

I would like to lose weight steadily   2   ☐

I would like to lose weight as fast as
safely possible   1   ☐ *2*

Your total: ☐ *2*

Now check your score
8–12
Your starting calorie level is 1,000 and your Set Diet is Diet
One; see page 103.

13–20
Your starting calorie level is 1,250 and your Set Diet is Diet
Two; see page 115.

21–30
Your starting calorie level is 1,500 and your Set Diet is Diet
Three; see page 126.

· YOUR SET DIET ·

On each of the three Set Diets, every day's eating for a
minimum of fourteen days is specified. There is still plenty
of choice, though, to ensure you will be eating the way you
like to eat. This diet will get your slimming off to a great
start because:
· It is easy to follow.

THE JUNK FOOD DIET

· When you're starting a diet, a set format helps bolster your determination.

· It gives you a sense of security.

· It shows you exactly what a varied diet is like, so when (and if) you switch to the Pick Your Own Plan, or a maintenance plan, you'll be better equipped.

When you have been on the Set Diet for a minimum of two weeks, you have a choice of action.

If you don't need to lose any more weight, turn to Chapter 11 and find out how to keep that weight off!

If you do need to lose more weight you can either continue with your Set Diet by returning to the beginning and repeating the fourteen days, or you can move to the Pick Your Own Plan. The choice is yours, but if you have more than a stone left to lose, I do recommend that you move to the Pick Your Own Plan, as it offers much more flexibility – you create your own diet without having to do anything other than select a menu to your personal calorie total, and there is the added bonus of 'eating out' and 'days off' schemes built in!

Even if you are on the Pick Your Own Plan, you can return to the Set Diet any time you like. You'll find more information about both Set Diets and Pick Your Own Plans at the start of Chapters 7 and 8.

What to expect when you start dieting

When you begin your diet, here's what will happen. The fourteen-day Set Diet could see you lose from 7 lb up to as much as a stone, depending on your starting weight (the more you need to lose and the taller you are, the greater your initial weight loss will be) and other personal factors.

In the first week, the loss will be largest of all, and the

reason is that when you first reduce your calorie intake, your body uses up its carbohydrate store and loses surplus water too. So if you lose, say, 5 lb in the first week, around half of this will be the weight of water and carbohydrate lost, and the rest will be fat. After a few more days of dieting, the fluid loss will stop and any more weight you lose will be pure fat. So in the second week, your weight loss will be smaller.

This is normal and correct, and not because the diet 'isn't working' or because you've done anything wrong. It is what happens to everyone.

As your diet progresses

When you've been slimming a while longer, you'll probably notice that you don't lose exactly the same amount every week, however carefully you have been sticking to your diet. This isn't anything to worry about either. For women in particular, weight loss fluctuation can be quite spectacular. Often in the first two weeks of their menstrual cycle, they lose a lot, mid-cycle they lose a steady amount and just before a period they may put weight on, no matter how carefully they've dieted. This weight gain is fluid, not fat, and it will go around the third day of the period.

Weight loss fluctuations from week to week, whatever your sex, don't really matter. What does matter is that over the course of, say, a month, you weigh less than you did the previous month. If over the course of a whole month, however, you don't lose a single pound (assuming you're not at your target weight yet, of course!) read on . . .

If your weight loss slows right down or stops

The nearer you get to your target weight, the more likely you are to find your weight loss slowing down. This *doesn't* necessarily mean that you have been cheating! There is a scientific explanation. The slimmer you are, the fewer calories your body needs to maintain its weight (that's why an 8-stone girl needs to eat less than a 15-stone man). So if, for instance, you now weigh 10 stone instead of your previous 13 stone, you will need to eat less to maintain your new weight – and less on your slimming diet to keep up a suitable calorie deficit.

This 'sticking point' often happens about two-thirds of the way down towards your target weight. Your weight loss slows down from, say, 2 lb a week to $\frac{1}{2}$ lb a week and then it stops altogether. Of course, everyone is different, and your own sticking point might be reached earlier, or later, or even not at all. It is certainly not going to happen while you are on your first fourteen-day Set Diet. But when it does happen, then you simply move *down* a calorie level. If, for example, you've been dieting on 1,500 calories a day, you move down to 1,250. If you've been on 1,250, you move to 1,000. If you are one of the minority who is already on the 1,000 calories a day diet, you can reduce to 900 a day by cutting out your daily 100-calorie treat *or* you can increase your body's calorie needs by stepping up your activity. You could burn up an extra 100 calories with, for example, a half-hour medium-paced walk, or a fifteen-minute cycle ride, or a ten-minute jog.

Ninety-nine per cent of dieters need never go below 1,000 calories a day to reach target weight, 50 per cent will never have to go below 1,250 and many will reach target still on 1,500. So don't worry too much about your sticking point until you get there.

And if you do get there, here's one other small thought. You've been on your diet a while. Are you checking out your portion sizes? In other words, is that 8-oz potato *really* an 8-oz potato, or is it 12 oz? Is that $\frac{1}{2}$ oz pat of butter nearer 1 oz? You need only a couple of portion mistakes on the generous side each day to tip the balance from steady weight loss to little or no weight loss. This is the most likely explanation of your problem if weight loss is very slow early on in your diet rather than towards the end. So before you do anything else, check it out.

If you lose weight too quickly

The calorie level we've chosen for you should result in a steady weight loss of anything up to 3 lb a week. But there are always exceptions that prove the rule. If (after the initial week's big weight loss) you are losing more than this, you might think about increasing your calorie level. The main problem with losing weight too quickly (discussed in more detail in Chapter 5) is that you may get hungry and give up your diet. So if you are losing weight quickly and feel hungry – especially if you were a borderline case in our questionnaire – step up to the next calorie band. Already on 1,500? A few people – mostly active men and teenagers or people with a lot of weight to lose – may find they can diet successfully on 1,600 or even more calories a day. If that happens to you, simply add 100 calories a day to your diet from the Pick Your Own snack listings on pages 188–94. Further on into your diet, for reasons already explained, you may need to lower your calorie level again.

· TIPS ·

The following dieting tips apply to *everyone* throughout their slimming campaign:

· Plan your day's eating well in advance when possible.

· Keep a diary and record how much you've eaten, what you ate, what you liked, your thoughts, etc. It helps.

· Drink plenty of calorie-free drinks: they help fill you up and keep your digestive system working well (for a list, see page 98).

· Eat everything you are allowed on your diet.

· Take your time over your food: research shows that slim people eat more slowly!

· RULES ·

Compulsory tips to help you get the most benefit from your diet! They also apply to everyone throughout the diet.

· Weigh yourself no more than once a week.

· Vary your meal choices as much as possible, aiming to have no main meal more than once a week.

· When cooking red meats, bacon, etc., cook until well done enough for most of the fat to run out. If making gravy or sauces, pour off surplus fat first.

· When frying use a non-stick pan and ensure oil is at the correct, high, temperature before adding food. Fry in corn, sunflower, safflower, rapeseed or olive oil; don't use lard.

· Remove visible fat from meat before cooking.

· Eat when you're hungry, not by the clock. If you ever get hungry between or after meals, and you don't have any snacks to spare, choose items from the unlimited list (opposite).

· Weigh or measure foods when amounts are stated.

· Don't waste calories. Never use a high-calorie ingredient in cooking or preparing food when a lower-calorie one would do just as well, and never eat anything you don't really want or need.

· If you have a day – or more – when your dieting gets off course, for whatever reason, don't let it tempt you to give up. For more detailed advice on coping with dieting disasters and problems, turn to Chapters 9 and 10.

Guidelines for sweet toothers

If you are choosing your treats calorie allowance in sweet items, follow these rules:

· Never eat your sweet treats when you are really hungry. Always satisfy hunger first, with a savoury food snack or meal within your diet, then have the sweet food.

· It is better to choose a single-item sweet food, such as a slice of cake or a chocolate bar, and eat it straight away in one go than pick a pack of chewy sweets or mints that will stay in your mouth over a long period.

· It is better to eat your sweet treat as part of a meal – say, as a dessert – than on its own.

· Clean your teeth after each sweet treat.

· Never go to bed at night without cleaning your teeth thoroughly.

· UNLIMITEDS ·

Quantities of all the following foods, drinks and seasonings are unlimited throughout your diet. That means that you can have them whenever you like, in reasonable amounts. The Eats will help fill you up, add colour and variety to your diet and help provide vital nutrients, in particular vitamin C. The Drinks will also help fill you up and help your digestive system. The Others will add taste and variety to your diet. However, none of the Unlimiteds is compulsory – with the obvious exception of your own choice of drinks, without which you would soon die! – so if you choose not to have them, you will still get a healthy, balanced, varied diet from the basic Junk Food Diet in the next chapters.

Drinks

Water, mineral water, soda water, calorie-free mixers and canned fizzy drinks, calorie-free squashes, PLJ, weak black tea, weak black coffee, herbal tea, lemon tea (unsweetened).

Eats

Lettuce, tomato, cress, onion, cucumber, cabbage, Chinese leaves, chicory, cauliflower, spring greens, pickled onion, carrot, celery, peppers (any colour), radish, beansprouts, mushrooms. All these can be raw or cooked without fat.

Others

Fresh or dried herbs and spices, oil-free French dressing, lemon juice, Worcestershire sauce, soya sauce, mustard, garlic, vinegar, lemon slices.

7 · THE JUNK FOOD DIET – 2

· THE SET DIETS ·

Before you begin the Set Diet that we decided was right for you in the last chapter, read through the following notes.

Breakfast

Every day there is a choice of two breakfasts. If you don't like breakfast at 'breakfast time', you can eat this meal anytime during the day as an extra snack. In fact, if you habitually don't eat breakfast, I strongly advise you not to start trying now. At least one of the breakfasts every day can be packed, so you could perhaps take it to work and eat it as a mid-morning snack.

The light meal

Most people will want to eat this around lunchtime, but if you happen to prefer your main meal at lunchtime, this will be your tea/supper. There is a choice of either a hot light meal or a cold one which can be packed for a working lunch – or you could eat it in the park, or in the canteen while you talk to your mates.

The main meal

There are four choices of main meal: a family choice of a recipe dish; a quick and easy meal suitable for singles, non-cooks and people in a hurry; the heat and serve alternative, which is a complete ready meal, usually with the addition of a vegetable or salad; and lastly there is a takeaway choice.

Snacks

Every day you choose two snacks. One is a choice of either milk (which you can use in drinks or as a drink on its own) or yogurt, the other is fruit.

The milk snack on all diets is ⅓ pint (200 ml) of skimmed milk, which can be used either in your tea or coffee or as a drink on its own. If you prefer your drinks black and don't like drinking milk, have a low-calorie diet fruit yogurt, such as Shape or Diet Ski, instead. (Ordinary fruit yogurts marked 'low fat' aren't particularly low in calories; look for a brand around 50 calories a tub.)

The fruit snack is one of the following fruits every day: 1 apple, 2 apricots, 4 oz (115 g) cherries, 5 oz (140 g) fruit salad, 4 oz (115 g) grapes, 1 grapefruit, 3 greengages, 2 mandarins, 4 oz (115 g) mango, average 6 oz (150 g) slice melon, 1 nectarine, 1 orange, 4 oz (115 g) papaya, 1 pear, 4 oz (115 g 2 rings) pineapple, 2 plums, 2 satsumas, 2 tangerines, 5 oz (140 g) any soft berry fruit, e.g. raspberries, strawberries or blackberries, 4 oz (115 g) any stewed fruit, e.g. apple or rhubarb, cooked either with sugar from your treats list, or sweetened with artificial sweetener.

Your fruit should be fresh if possible, or frozen as a good alternative. If you use canned now and then, drain it of the syrup or juice it's in and weigh it or measure it out then. If for any reason one day you can't get your fruit supply, have instead 4 fl. oz (120 ml) fruit juice (longlife will do) or 1 oz (30 g) dried, 'no need to soak', apricots, peaches or prunes . . . that's about four pieces of dried fruit.

Treats/extras

Every day you can choose a Treat or an extra: 100, 200 or 300 calories' worth a day, depending on which diet level you are on.

Treats can be either sweet, such as cake, biscuits, desserts and chocolate, or alcohol, or savoury, such as bread and butter or crisps instead. They can be eaten as a dessert or as a snack whenever you like during the day. If you're choosing sweet treats, follow the tips on page 97 in Chapter 6.

Instead of a treat, you could choose an extra: an addition to your meal, for instance, such as extra chips, rice, or mayonnaise, or butter on your baked potato. It's up to you how you spend this treats allowance. Full lists of the allowed treats and extras appear on pages 184–94.

Unlimiteds

Don't forget to make the most of your unlimiteds – the foods, drinks and sundries listed in Chapter 6 that will help broaden your diet's horizons.

The Sunday brunch alternative

There are two sorts of Sunday eaters: those who have a lightish breakfast, a big lunch (probably a traditional one) and a tea or supper, and those who have a late combined breakfast/lunch (probably a fry-up), then a main meal in the evening. Decide which pattern you prefer and follow the appropriate Sunday diet.

Salad

Salad items are mentioned as accompaniments with some

light and main meals. If you don't like the items mentioned, pick an alternative from the Unlimited lists. When simply 'salad' is mentioned, choose whatever you like from the list in whatever quantity. If you're a total salad hater and follow the diet without any of these items, make doubly sure to eat all fruit and fruit juice allowed on the diet and get your full quota of vegetables mentioned. If you choose the takeaway frequently, this advice is even more important.

Bread

You choose which kind of bread you prefer. Softgrain white is an ideal compromise: it's high in calcium like all white bread, but with more fibre than ordinary white.

Milk

Your daily snack and cereal milk should be skimmed, but if you refuse to drink skimmed milk, semi-skimmed will only add an extra 20–30 calories a day to your diet. Full-cream milk is a terrible waste of calories in my opinion, but if you must have it, you can choose it as all or part of your daily Treat/Extra.

Frying

Here are some notes on the frying methods used in the Junk Food Diet.

Dry-frying: Use a good heavy non-stick pan. Wipe the bottom with a smear of oil on kitchen paper. Heat the pan. With eggs, add them to a *hot* pan. With fatty meat such as bacon add to a warm pan and gradually increase the heat until the fat runs out and the bacon (or whatever) cooks in its own fat. Always drain off any fat left in the pan at the end of cooking and pat the food dry on kitchen paper.

Stir-frying: Use a good non-stick pan or wok. Add one or

two teaspoons of oil and turn heat up high. Add shredded or stripped vegetables, meat, etc., as instructed, and stir constantly until food is just cooked. Add stock or water, not extra oil, if food gets too dry.

Shallow- or deep-frying: Make sure the oil is very hot before adding the food. Don't overfry. Remove food on a slatted spatula or spoon on to kitchen paper and drain thoroughly. Never refry fried foods to reheat them. They'll absorb twice as much fat.

Chips: Whenever oven chips are mentioned in the diet, you could substitute very thick-cut deep-fried chips instead – e.g. Beefeaters or home-made.

Finally . . .

Start the diet on a Monday. Make sure you have everything you need beforehand. Don't swop meals from different days around.

· DIET ONE ·
1,000 calories a day

Every day:

You may have Unlimiteds from the list on page 97.

You should have your two Snacks – your milk or yogurt and your fruit.

You can pick Treats/Extras up to 100 calories a day from the 50- and 100-calorie lists on pages 189–94.

DAY 1

Breakfast
EITHER 1 medium slice bread with a little low-fat spread

and 2 teaspoons of reduced-sugar jam or marmalade; 1 diet fruit yogurt; 4 fl oz (120 ml) unsweetened orange, grapefruit or pineapple juice

OR 1 oz (30 g) breakfast cereal of choice with 4 fl oz (120 ml) milk and 1 teaspoon sugar; 4 fl oz (120 ml) unsweetened orange, grapefruit or pineapple juice.

Light meal

EITHER 1 Birds Eye Chicken and Mushroom Casserole with 5 oz (140 g) instant mashed potato, 1 tomato

OR 1 Lean Cuisine Chicken and Prawn Cantonese with Noodles

OR 3 rye crispbreads or 1 mini pitta bread, filled with a mixture of 3 oz (85 g) cold cooked chicken or turkey, chopped, 1 level tablespoon reduced-calorie mayonnaise, chopped tomato and green pepper, 1 tablespoon sweetcorn; 1 apple.

Main meal

Family Choice: 1 portion Quick Boston Baked Beans (see recipe page 280) with 3 tablespoons mashed potato.

Quick and Easy: 2 large pork or beef sausages, well grilled or fried, or 1 pork chop, 4 tablespoons baked beans and 4 tablespoons instant mashed potato or 2 oz (55 g) oven chips, grilled.

Heat and Serve: 1 × 8 oz (225 g) can Heinz Beans with Sausages, 1 medium slice bread with a little low-fat spread.

Takeaway: EITHER 1 Spud U Like Spud 'n One, Sausage 'n Beans variety

OR 1 Wimpy Beanburger.

DAY 2

Breakfast

EITHER 2 medium slices bread with a little low-fat spread

and 3 teaspoons reduced-sugar jam or marmalade, ½ grapefruit or 4 oz (115 g) canned grapefruit segments

OR 2 Weetabix or Shredded Wheat, 1 teaspoon sugar, 5 fl oz (150 ml) milk, ½ grapefruit or 4 oz (115 g) canned grapefruit segments.

Light meal

EITHER 1 size-3 egg, dry-fried, 3 oz (85 g) oven chips

OR 2 size-3 eggs, scrambled, on 1 medium slice toast

OR 2 medium slices bread with a little low-fat spread, 1 hard-boiled egg, 1 teaspoon reduced-calorie mayonnaise, tomato and cress garnish.

Main meal

Family Choice: 1 portion Cottage Pie (see recipe page 272), 4 oz (115 g) mixed peas and carrots.

Quick and Easy: 2 frozen minced beef crispy pancakes, dry-fried, 3 oz (85 g) oven chips or 4 tablespoons instant mash, 1 tomato.

Heat and Serve: EITHER 1 individual Shepherds

OR Cottage pie

OR Spaghetti Bolognese, all with side salad.

Takeaway: EITHER 1 doner kebab

OR 1 Quarterpounder (McDonald's)

OR 1 Kingsize hamburger (Wimpy).

DAY 3

Breakfast

EITHER 1 medium slice bread with a little low-fat spread, 1 boiled egg, 4 fl oz (120 ml) unsweetened orange, grapefruit or pineapple juice

OR 1 medium slice bread with a little low-fat spread and 2 teaspoons reduced-sugar jam or marmalade, 1 banana.

Light meal

EITHER 1 large Frankfurter (hot dog), heated, in 1 soft finger roll with 2 oz (50 g) stir-fried onion slices and 1 dessertspoon sauce or relish of choice

OR 2 medium slices toast or 4 rye crispbreads with a little low-fat spread, 2 oz (55 g) light liver pâté, salad garnish.

Main meal

Family Choice: 1 portion Macaroni Cheese (see recipe page 265), 3 oz (85 g) green beans or large side salad.

Quick and Easy: 1 × 5 oz (140 g) slice mushroom or onion quiche, 3 oz (85 g) green beans, 1 tomato.

Heat and Serve: EITHER 1 Findus Dinner Supreme Lasagne OR 1 Birds Eye Mariner's Pasta Gratin, both with 3 oz (85 g) green beans or large side salad.

Takeaway: 1 Pizza Hut individual Sauce and Cheese Thin and Crispy pizza (no treat allowed today if you choose this takeaway).

DAY 4

Breakfast

As Day 1.

Light meal

EITHER 8 oz (225 g) baked potato with 3 tablespoons baked beans

OR 1 pitta bread filled with 1 chopped hard-boiled egg and salad items of choice plus oil-free dressing.

Main meal

Family Choice: EITHER 1 portion Beef Stir Fry (see recipe page 274), 5 tablespoons boiled rice or noodles

OR 1 portion Lamb Kebabs (see recipe page 277) with 3 tablespoons rice or noodles.

Quick and Easy: 4 oz (115 g) beefburger or Prizesteak, well grilled or fried, 2 oz (50 g) oven chips or 2 croquette potatoes, grilled or baked, 3 tablespoons peas or 1 small tub coleslaw in reduced-calorie vinaigrette.

Heat and Serve: EITHER 1 Findus Dinner Supreme Beef Teriyaki or Japonais

OR 1 McCain Continental Beef Platter, all with side salad.

Takeaway: As Day 2.

DAY 5

Breakfast

As Day 2.

Light meal

EITHER 2 size-3 eggs made into omelette, cooked in 1 teaspoon butter in non-stick pan, 1 waffle or potato cake, dry-fried, 1 tomato

OR 1 average Scotch egg with a large mixed salad.

Main meal

Family Choice: 1 portion Fisherman's Pie (see recipe page 258), 4 tablespoons sweetcorn or peas, 4 oz (115 g) broccoli or green beans.

Quick and Easy: EITHER 6 oz (170 g) fillet of white fish with 1 portion cheese sauce (see recipe page 251), 3 tablespoons instant mash, 4 tablespoons sweetcorn or peas

OR 4 fish fingers, grilled, 4 tablespoons instant mash and 4 tablespoons peas or baked beans.

Heat and Serve: 1 Birds Eye Captain's Pie, 4 oz (115 g) broccoli or green beans or mixed salad.

Takeaway: EITHER 1 McDonald's Filet-O-Fish

OR 1 Wimpy Fish and Chips (no treat allowed today if you choose this takeaway).

DAY 6

Breakfast

EITHER 1 × 3½ oz (100 g) can soft cod's roes on 1 medium slice toast with a little low-fat spread, 4 fl oz (120 ml) unsweetened orange, grapefruit or pineapple juice

OR 1 small slice bread with a little low-fat spread and 1 teaspoon reduced-sugar marmalade or jam, 1 Weetabix or Shredded Wheat with 4 fl oz (120 ml) milk.

Light meal

EITHER 5-in cheese and tomato pizza, grilled, mixed salad

OR 2 oz (55 g) reduced-fat Cheddar-style cheese with 3 cream crackers or 1½ oz (45 g) French bread with a little low-fat spread, salad.

Main meal

Family Choice: EITHER 1 portion Chicken Tikka (see recipe page 262) with 5 tablespoons boiled rice, tomato salad

OR 1 portion Chicken Supreme (see recipe page 261), 4 tablespoons boiled rice or 5 tablespoons mashed potato, 3 oz (85 g) green beans.

Quick and Easy: 1 average chicken breast portion or crunch-coated chicken escalope, grilled or baked, 4 oz (115 g) boiled or baked potato, 3 tablespoons sweetcorn or peas.

Heat and Serve: 1 Findus Chicken Supreme, salad.

Takeaway: EITHER 1 chicken chow mein

OR 1 portion Tandoori chicken PLUS 1 chapati or ½ portion plain rice with either takeaway (no treat allowed today if you choose either of these takeaways).

DAY 7

Breakfast

EITHER 6 oz (170 g) smoked haddock, 1 size-3 poached egg, ¼ oz (7 g) butter, 1 small slice bread

OR 2 oz (55 g) crisply cooked lean bacon or ham, 4 oz (115 g) sliced mushrooms, stir-fried

OR 1 dry-fried egg, 1 small slice bread

OR as Day 1.

Light meal

EITHER 1 × 10 oz (285 g) can thick pea and ham soup, 1 medium slice bread

OR 1 × 4 oz (115 g) slice quiche, 1 small tub coleslaw in reduced-calorie mayonnaise.

Main meal

Family Choice: 3 oz (85 g) well-done lean roast beef, leg of lamb or pork, 1 large chunk roast potato or 4 oz (115 g) boiled potatoes, 4 oz (115 g) broccoli or green beans or cauliflower, 4 oz (115 g) carrots, 1 tablespoon gravy from stock cube, 4 oz (115 g) stewed or soft fruit.

Quick and Easy: 4 oz (115 g) beefburger, grilled, 3 oz (85 g) oven chips or 1 burger bun, 2 oz (50 g) sweetcorn or side salad, 1 teaspoon relish.

Heat and Serve: 1 Birds Eye Roast Beef Platter.

Takeaway: EITHER 1 doner kebab

OR 1 Spud U Like Spud 'n One, Savoury Mince variety.

Sunday brunch exchange

If you prefer, have the following brunch *instead* of both the Day 7 breakfast and the light meal. (So you have just a brunch and a main meal today.) 1 size-3 egg, fried, 1 chipolata or 1 good slice black pudding, well fried or grilled, 1 potato cake, dry-fried or grilled, 1 back rasher, well grilled, 3 tablespoons baked beans or 2 tablespoons dry-fried mushrooms, 1 medium slice bread with a little low-fat spread, 1 dessertspoon sauce of choice.

DAY 8

Breakfast

As Day 1.

Light meal

EITHER 2 oz (55 g) corned beef or 3 oz (85 g) leftover roast meat, 2 croquette potatoes or 2 oz (55 g) oven chips, 1 tomato

OR 2 medium slices bread with a little low-fat spread, 1½ oz (45 g) corned beef or 2 oz (55 g) cold roast meat, 1 dessertspoon pickle, salad.

Main meal

Family Choice: 4 oz (115 g) lean boiled gammon with 1 portion Parsley Sauce (see recipe page 251), 3 oz (85 g) boiled potatoes, 3 oz (85 g) broad beans or 5 oz (140 g) broccoli.

Quick and Easy: 4 oz (115 g) bacon steak, well grilled, with 1 portion parsley sauce from packet mix, 4 oz (115 g) boiled or instant mash potatoes, 3 oz (85 g) broad beans or sweetcorn.

Heat and Serve: 1 Birds Eye Menu Master Gammon Steak Platter, salad.

Takeaway: 1 portion barbecued spare ribs.

DAY 9

Breakfast

As Day 2.

Light meal

EITHER 1 portion boil-in-bag fish in butter sauce, 3 tablespoons instant mash, 4 oz (115 g) green beans

OR 2 medium slices bread with low-fat spread, 1 × 3½ oz (100 g) can tuna in brine or oil, well-drained, salad, 1 dessertspoon salad cream or 1 teaspoon mayonnaise.

Main meal

Family Choice: EITHER 1 portion Basic Mince (see recipe page 270), 4 oz (115 g) boiled or mashed potatoes or 3 oz (85 g) boiled rice, 3 oz (85 g) peas

OR 1 portion Chilli con Carne (see recipe page 271), 2 oz (55 g) boiled rice.

Quick and Easy: 1 pack Ross Beef Stir Fry (any variety) cooked as instructed, salad.

Heat and Serve: 1 individual pack Birds Eye or Sainsbury's Chilli con Carne with Rice, salad.

Takeaway: 1 Spud U Like Spud 'n One, Chilli con Carne variety without butter.

DAY 10

Breakfast

As Day 3.

Light meal

EITHER 1 size-3 egg, dry-fried, 2 slices streaky bacon, well grilled or fried until crisp, 2 oz (55 g) mushrooms, stir-fried, 1 tomato

OR 2 medium slices bread with a little low-fat spread, 2 slices very lean ham, salad garnish, 1 teaspoon salad cream or mustard.

Main meal

Family Choice: EITHER 1 portion Risotto (see recipe page 269), salad

OR 1 portion Scampi Provençale (see recipe page 259), 6 tablespoons boiled rice, salad.

Quick and Easy: 2 chicken and mushroom or chicken curry crispy pancakes, dry-fried or grilled, 4 tablespoons instant mash, 3 tablespoons sweetcorn.

Heat and Serve: EITHER 1 Birds Eye Prawn Curry

OR 1 Findus Kashmiri Chicken Curry with Rice, both with salad.

Takeaway: EITHER 1 chicken chow mein

OR 1 Spud U Like Spud 'n One, Chicken Curry variety, no butter.

DAY 11

Breakfast

As Day 4.

Light meal

EITHER 2 oz (55 g) reduced-fat Cheddar-style cheese, melted on 1 medium slice toast topped with sliced tomato

OR 2 mini pittas or 1 large pitta filled with 2 tablespoons half-fat cream cheese, chopped vegetables of choice (e.g. peppers, tomato, onion), 1 tablespoon sweetcorn, 2 black olives (optional).

Main meal

Family Choice: EITHER 1 portion Beef Goulash (see recipe page 273)

OR 1 portion Beef Stroganoff (see recipe page 274), both with 4 tablespoons boiled rice, 3 tablespoons peas or 4 oz (115 g) broccoli.

Quick and Easy: 4 oz (115 g) beefburger, well grilled, 3 oz (85 g) oven chips, grilled, 1 tomato.

Heat and Serve: 1 Birds Eye Beef Stew and Dumplings, 3 oz (85 g) green beans or salad.

Takeaway: Chinese beef and green peppers in oyster sauce, ½ portion plain rice (no treat allowed today if you choose this takeaway).

DAY 12

Breakfast

As Day 5.

Light meal

EITHER 1 × 10 oz (285 g) can cream of chicken soup, 1 medium roll, low-fat spread

OR 1 medium slice bread with a little low-fat spread, 2 lean slices chicken, turkey or ham, 1 small tub coleslaw in reduced-calorie dressing.

Main meal

Family Choice: EITHER 1 portion Cod Creole (see recipe page 259), 6 oz (170 g) baked potato or 6 tablespoons boiled rice

OR 1 portion Tuna Florentino (see recipe page 257).

Quick and Easy: 1 haddock or cod steak (frozen) in light and crispy batter, grilled or baked, 3 oz (85 g) oven chips, 3 tablespoons peas.

Heat and Serve: 1 McCain Scampi and Chips.

Takeaway: Chinese king prawns and mushrooms, ½ portion boiled rice (no treat allowed today if you choose this takeaway).

DAY 13

Breakfast

As Day 6.

Light meal

EITHER 1 × 7½ oz (210 g) can macaroni cheese, 1 small slice bread, 1 tomato

OR 2 oz (55 g) Brie cheese, 2 cream crackers or crispbreads with a little low-fat spread, salad.

Main meal

Family Choice: 3 chipolata sausages, well cooked or 1 chipolata and 1 size-3 egg, dry-fried, 3 oz (85 g) oven chips or 2 potato cakes, dry-fried or grilled, 3 tablespoons baked beans or peas.

Quick and Easy: As Family Choice.

Heat and Serve: 1 Findus Toad in the Hole, 3 tablespoons baked beans or peas.

Takeaway: 1 Pizza Hut Thin and Crispy pizza (no treat allowed today if you choose this takeaway).

DAY 14

Breakfast

As Day 7.

Light meal

EITHER 1 × 10½ oz (300 g) can Heinz Farmhouse Vegetable soup, 1 average roll

OR 1 small tin tuna or salmon, well drained, 1 medium slice bread with a little low-fat spread, salad.

Main meal

Family Choice: 4 oz (115 g) lean roast chicken or turkey, 1 large chunk roast potato or 4 oz (115 g) boiled potato, 2 tablespoons peas, 4 oz (115 g) carrots, 2 tablespoons gravy from stock cube, 1 dessertspoon stuffing.

Quick and Easy: 1 average chicken portion, hot or cold, plain or with Tandoori coating, 1 small tub rice salad or 4 oz (115 g) boiled potatoes, salad.

Heat and Serve: EITHER 1 Birds Eye Roast Turkey Platter
OR 1 McCain Sweet and Sour Chicken, salad.

Takeaway: 1 portion Kentucky Fried Chicken with barbecue beans and coleslaw.

Sunday brunch exchange

As Day 7.

· DIET TWO ·
1,250 calories a day

Every day:

You may have Unlimiteds from the list on page 97.

You should have two Snacks — your milk or yogurt and your fruit.

You can pick Treats/Extras up to 200 calories a day from the 50-, 100-, 150- and 200-calorie lists on pages 189–94.

DAY 1

Breakfast

EITHER 1 medium slice bread with a little low-fat spread and 2 teaspoons reduced-sugar jam or marmalade, 1 diet fruit yogurt, 4 fl oz (120 ml) unsweetened orange, grapefruit or pineapple juice

OR 1 oz (30 g) breakfast cereal of choice with 4 fl oz (120 ml) milk and 1 teaspoon sugar, 4 fl oz (120 ml) unsweetened orange, grapefruit or pineapple juice.

Light meal

EITHER 2 chicken and bacon crispy pancakes, dry-fried, 3 tablespoons sweetcorn, 1 small slice bread with a little low-fat spread

OR 1 medium cooked chicken portion or 4 oz (115 g) leftover chicken meat, 1 large salad or 1 small tub coleslaw in reduced-calorie dressing, 1 small slice bread with a little low-fat spread.

Main meal

Family Choice: 1 portion Toad in the Hole (see recipe page 280), 3 tablespoons baked beans.

Quick and Easy: 2 large pork or beef sausages, well grilled, 5 tablespoons instant mashed potato, 3 tablespoons baked beans.

Heat and Serve: 1 Findus Toad in the Hole, 3 tablespoons baked beans or 1 large salad.

Takeaway: 1 Spud U Like Spud 'n One, Sausage and Beans variety, including butter.

DAY 2

Breakfast

EITHER 2 medium slices bread with a little low-fat spread and 3 tablespoons reduced-sugar jam or marmalade, $\frac{1}{2}$ grapefruit or 4 oz (115 g) canned grapefruit segments

OR 2 Weetabix or Shredded Wheat, 1 teaspoon sugar, $\frac{1}{4}$ pint (150 ml) milk, $\frac{1}{2}$ grapefruit or 4 oz (115 g) canned grapefruit segments.

Light meal

EITHER 1$\frac{1}{2}$ oz (45 g) Cheddar cheese, melted, on 1 medium slice toast spread with a little low-fat spread, topped with 1 sliced tomato, salad garnish

OR 1$\frac{1}{2}$ oz (45 g) Cheddar cheese with 1 medium slice bread or 2 cream crackers and a little low-fat spread, 1 dessertspoon pickle of choice and 1 tomato, salad garnish.

Main meal

Family Choice: portion Corned Beef Hash (see recipe page 279), 3 tablespoons sweetcorn, 2 oz (55 g) green beans.

Quick and Easy: 4 × 1 oz (30 g) slices corned beef, 1 × 4 oz

(115 g) carton Shape potato salad, large mixed salad, 1 dessertspoon pickle of choice, 1 banana.

Heat and Serve: 1 Findus Dinner Supreme Beef Madras, 1 dessertspoon chutney of choice, tomato salad.

Takeaway: EITHER 1 doner kebab

OR 1 Quarterpounder (McDonald's)

OR 1 Kingsize (Wimpy).

DAY 3

Breakfast

EITHER 1 medium slice bread with a little low-fat spread, 1 boiled egg, 4 fl oz (120 ml) unsweetened orange, grapefruit or pineapple juice

OR 1 medium slice bread with a little low-fat spread and 2 teaspoons reduced-sugar jam or marmalade, 1 banana or diet yogurt.

Light meal

EITHER 1 × 10½ oz (300 g) can Heinz Tomato and Lentil or Pea and Ham soup, 1 medium slice bread with a little low-fat spread, 1 diet yogurt or 1 apple

OR 3 oz (85 g) very lean ham or 2 oz (55 g) pâté of choice, 1 medium slice bread with little low-fat spread, tomato salad.

Main meal

Family Choice: 1 portion Spanish Omelette (see recipe page 256), 2 oz (55 g) oven chips, 4 tablespoons peas.

Quick and Easy: 2 size-3 eggs, dry-fried, 4 oz (115 g) oven chips, 4 tablespoons peas.

Heat and Serve: 1 individual cheese and onion or mushroom quiche, large salad or 3 tablespoons sweetcorn salad.

Takeaway: EITHER 1 Spud U Like Spud 'n One, Egg and Cheese variety

OR 1 individual cheese and tomato pizza.

DAY 4

Breakfast

As Day 1.

Light meal

EITHER 1 × 8 oz (225 g) can baked beans in tomato or barbecue sauce on 1 medium slice toast with a little low-fat spread, 1 apple

OR 1 × 3½ oz (100 g) tin of tuna, well drained, 1 average bread roll or 2 small slices bread with a little low-fat spread, 1 × 4 oz (115 g) tub Shape salad, any variety except potato, salad garnish.

Main meal

Family Choice: 1 portion Spaghetti Bolognese (see recipe page 267), salad.

Quick and Easy: 4 oz (115 g) beefburger, well grilled or dry-fried, 4 oz (115 g) oven chips, 4 tablespoons peas or sweetcorn or baked beans.

Heat and Serve: EITHER 1 Birds Eye Spaghetti Bolognese with 1 dessertspoon Parmesan cheese

OR 1 Birds Eye Lasagne, 1 orange.

Takeaway: 1 regular hamburger with regular French fries.

DAY 5

Breakfast

As Day 2.

Light meal

EITHER 2 size-3 eggs, poached or scrambled with ¼ oz (7 g) butter on 1 medium slice toast with a little low-fat spread

OR 1 Scotch egg with large salad, 1 teaspoon mayonnaise or dressing of choice.

Main meal

Family Choice: 1 portion Monkfish Kebabs (see recipe page 260), 5 tablespoons boiled rice, salad.

Quick and Easy: 4 fish fingers, grilled or dry-fried, 5 tablespoons instant mash, 3 tablespoons peas or baked beans, 1 banana.

Heat and Serve: 1 individual cod crumble, salad.

Takeaway: Wimpy Fish and Chips.

DAY 6

Breakfast

EITHER 1 × 3½ oz (100 g) can soft cod's roes on 1 medium slice toast with a little low-fat spread, 4 fl oz (120 ml) unsweetened orange, grapefruit or pineapple juice

OR 1 small slice bread with a little low-fat spread and 1 teaspoon reduced-sugar jam or marmalade, 1 Weetabix or Shredded Wheat with 4 fl oz (120 ml) milk.

Light meal

EITHER 1 Pizza Toast (see recipe page 254) or 1 Findus French Bread pizza, any variety, salad

OR Ploughman's Lunch — 1½ oz (45 g) Cheddar cheese or 3 oz (85 g) reduced-fat Cheddar-style cheese, 1½ oz (45 g) French bread or 1 large slice bread with a little low-fat spread, 1 dessertspoon pickle, salad garnish.

Main meal

Family Choice: 1 portion Chicken Curry (see recipe page 263), 6 tablespoons boiled rice, 1 grilled poppadom or 1 dessertspoon chutney of choice.

Quick and Easy: 2 chicken curry crispy pancakes, dry-fried, 4 oz (115 g) oven chips, 4 oz (115 g) green beans or broccoli.

Heat and Serve: 1 Findus Dinner Supreme Chicken Korma, 1 poppadom or 1 dessertspoon chutney of choice.
Takeaway: 1 chicken chow mein plus ½ portion plain rice.

DAY 7

Breakfast

EITHER 6 oz (170 g) smoked haddock, 1 size-3 egg, poached, ¼ oz (7 g) butter, 1 small slice bread

OR 2 oz (55 g) crisply cooked lean bacon or ham, 4 oz (115 g) sliced mushrooms, stir-fried, or 1 dry-fried size-3 egg, 1 small slice bread

OR as Day 1.

Light meal

EITHER 1 × 10½ oz (300 g) can cream of tomato soup, 1 average bread roll or 2 small slices bread, 1 apple

OR 1 × 3½ oz (100 g) can salmon or sardines or tuna, well drained, 1 average bread roll or 2 small slices bread, little low-fat spread, salad.

Main meal

Family Choice: 4 oz (115 g) lean well-done roast beef, leg of lamb or pork, 6 oz (170 g) baked potato or 2 small chunks roast potato, 4 oz (115 g) greens or cauliflower or carrots, 3 tablespoons peas, 2 teaspoons mint, horseradish or apple sauce, 2 tablespoons gravy from stock cube, 5 oz (140 g) stewed or soft fruit with 1 tablespoon single cream.

Quick and Easy: 1 individual steak and kidney or beef and onion pie, 3 tablespoons instant mash, 3 tablespoons peas and carrots.

Heat and Serve: 1 Birds Eye Roast Beef Platter or Prize-steak Platter, 1 banana or French-style yogurt.

Takeaway: As Day 4.

Sunday brunch exchange

If you prefer, have the following brunch *instead* of both the Day 7 breakfast and the light meal. (So you have just a brunch and main meal today.)

1 size-3 egg, fried, 2 chipolatas or 2 good slices black pudding, well fried or grilled, 1 potato cake, dry-fried or grilled, 1 back rasher, well grilled, 3 tablespoons baked beans or 2 tablespoons dry-fried mushrooms, 1 medium slice bread with a little low-fat spread, 1 dessertspoon sauce of choice.

DAY 8

Breakfast

As Day 1.

Light meal

EITHER 3 oz (85 g) leftover roast meat, lean only, or lean boiled ham or tongue, 1 medium slice bread with a little low-fat spread, 1 small tub coleslaw in reduced-calorie dressing, salad

OR 1 × 8 oz (225 g) can baked beans in barbecue sauce or tomato sauce on 1 medium slice toast with a little low-fat spread and either 1 oz (30 g) reduced-fat Cheddar-style cheese grated over top or 1 tub diet yogurt.

Main meal

Family Choice: 1 portion Tagliatelle with Ham (see recipe page 266), salad.

Quick and Easy: 4 oz (115 g) gammon or bacon steak, 4 oz (115 g) oven chips or 6 oz (170 g) baked potato with ¼ oz (7 g) butter, 4 tablespoons peas or broad beans.

Heat and Serve: EITHER 1 McCain Oven Meal Gammon and Chips

OR 1 Birds Eye Gammon Steak Platter, both with salad, 1

apple PLUS extra 100 calories' worth of any Extra (see pages 189–92)

Takeaway: EITHER 1 portion barbecued spare ribs plus $\frac{1}{2}$ portion plain rice

OR 1 doner kebab.

DAY 9

Breakfast

As Day 2.

Light Meal

EITHER 5-in cheese and tomato pizza with 1 oz (30 g) extra Cheddar cheese grated on, salad

OR Ploughman's, as Day 6.

Main meal

Family Choice: EITHER 1 portion Basic Mince (see recipe page 270), 5 tablespoons mashed potato, 4 oz (115 g) green beans

OR 1 portion Chilli con Carne (see recipe page 271), 6 tablespoons boiled rice, salad.

Quick and Easy: EITHER 4 oz (115 g) steak grill or 2 chilli beef crispy pancakes, dry-fried, 4 tablespoons instant mash, 4 oz (115 g) green beans

OR $\frac{1}{2}$ can Campbell's Chilli con Carne with 4 tablespoons boiled rice, salad.

Heat and Serve: 1 Birds Eye Chilli con Carne with Rice, salad.

Takeaway: Spud U Like Spud 'n One, Chilli con Carne variety, with butter.

DAY 10

Breakfast

As Day 3.

Light meal

EITHER 1 size-3 egg, dry-fried, 3 oz (85 g) oven chips or 3 croquette potatoes, 1 tomato

OR 1 size-3 egg, hard-boiled, 2 medium slices bread with a little low-fat spread, salad, 2 teaspoons mayonnaise.

Main meal

Family Choice: 1 portion Sweet and Sour Pork (see recipe page 277), 4 tablespoons boiled rice or 3 oz (85 g) boiled noodles, salad.

Quick and Easy: 1 average trimmed pork chop, grilled, 3 croquette potatoes or 4 oz (115 g) savoury noodles, 4 tablespoons peas or 4 oz (115 g) broccoli, 1 portion Barbecue Sauce (see recipe page 252) or 2 tablespoons stuffing from packet.

Heat and Serve: 1 McCain Sweet and Sour Chicken with Rice, 1 spring roll or 1 banana, salad.

Takeaway: 1 Kentucky Fried Chicken Dinner for One with beans and chips (but choose only 100-calories' worth of treats today if you pick this takeaway).

DAY 11

Breakfast

As Day 4.

Light meal

EITHER 3 fish fingers, grilled, 3 tablespoons mashed potato, 4 tablespoons peas or baked beans

OR 1 × 3½ oz (100 g) can tuna, sardines or salmon, well drained, 1 medium slice bread with a little low-fat spread, salad, 2 teaspoons mayonnaise.

Main meal

Family Choice: 3 pork or beef chipolata sausages, well

grilled or fried, 1 size-3 egg, dry-fried, 4 oz (115 g) oven chips.

Quick and Easy: As Family Choice.

Heat and Serve: 1 Bejam or Asda Sausage and Mash.

Takeaway: 1 Wimpy Bacon in a Bun.

DAY 12

Breakfast

As Day 5.

Light meal

EITHER Cauliflower cheese − 10 oz (285 g) lightly cooked cauliflower topped with 1 portion Cheese Sauce (see recipe page 251) with 1 oz (30 g) extra Cheddar cheese grated over top and browned under grill, salad

OR 1½ oz (45 g) Cheddar cheese or 2 oz (55 g) Edam or Brie with 3 cream crackers or crispbreads, a little low-fat spread, 1 dessertspoon pickle of choice, 1 tomato.

Main meal

Family Choice: 1 portion Tuna Florentino (see recipe page 257), 4 oz (115 g) boiled potatoes, salad.

Quick and Easy: 2 fish cakes, dry-fried, or 1 oven crispy cod steak (battered), 4 oz (115 g) oven chips or potato bites, 4 tablespoons peas or sweetcorn.

Heat and Serve: EITHER 1 Birds Eye Oven Crispy Fish and Chips

OR 1 McCain Cod and Chips.

Takeaway: EITHER 1 Wimpy Fish and Chips

OR 1 McDonald's Filet-O-Fish.

DAY 13

Breakfast

As Day 6.

Light meal

EITHER 2 oz (55 g) beefburger, well grilled or fried, 2 croquette potatoes, 4 tablespoons baked beans, 1 teaspoon relish

OR 4 oz (115 g) very lean ham, 1 average bread roll with a little low-fat spread, salad, 1 teaspoon dressing of choice.

Main meal

Family Choice: EITHER 1 portion Moussaka (see recipe page 271)

OR 1 portion Beef Enchiladas (see recipe page 272), salad. Quick and Easy: 3 Mexican taco shells, cooked as instructed and filled with ½ can beef taco filling, topped with taco sauce and chopped salad items of choice.

Heat and Serve: 1 Findus Moussaka, salad.

Takeaway: EITHER 1 Pizza Hut Lasagne

OR 1 Pizza Hut Spaghetti Bolognese

OR 1 McDonald's Quarterpounder.

DAY 14

Breakfast

As Day 7.

Light Meal

EITHER 1 French Bread pizza, any variety, salad

OR 2 oz (55 g) liver pâté, 3 crispbreads or 2 small slices bread with low-fat spread, salad, 1 apple.

Main meal

Family Choice: 4 oz (115 g) roast chicken or turkey, 2 small chunks roast potato or 6 oz (170 g) baked potato, 4 oz (115 g) mixed peas and carrots, 4 oz (115 g) broccoli or sprouts, 2 tablespoons thin gravy, 2 tablespoons packet stuffing.

Quick and Easy: 1 average roast chicken or Tandoori

chicken portion, 5 tablespoons instant mash or 6 oz (170 g) baked potato or 2 small slices bread with little low-fat spread or 3 oz (85 g) oven chips, 3 tablespoons peas or sweetcorn, salad.

Heat and Serve: EITHER 1 Birds Eye Roast Chicken Platter

OR 1 Birds Eye Roast Turkey Platter, both with 1 banana or diet yogurt.

Takeaway: EITHER 6 McDonald's Chicken McNuggets and regular French fries

OR 1 Wimpy Chicken in a Bun.

Sunday brunch exchange

As Day 7.

· DIET THREE ·
1,500 calories a day

Every day:

You may have Unlimiteds from the list on page 97.

You should have your two Snacks – your milk or yogurt and your fruit.

You can pick Treats/Extras up to 300 calories a day from the 50-, 100-, 150-, 200- and 300-calorie lists on pages 189–94.

DAY 1

Breakfast

EITHER 1 large slice or 2 small slices bread with a little low-fat spread and 2 teaspoons reduced-sugar jam or marmalade, 1 diet fruit yogurt, 4 fl oz (120 ml) unsweetened orange, grapefruit or pineapple juice

OR 1½ oz (45 g) breakfast cereal of choice with ¼ pint (150 ml) milk and 1 teaspoon sugar, 4 fl oz (120 ml) unsweetened orange, grapefruit or pineapple juice.

Light meal

EITHER 2 chicken and bacon crispy pancakes, dry-fried, 4 tablespoons sweetcorn, 1 medium slice bread with little low-fat spread

OR 1 medium cooked chicken portion or 4 oz (115 g) leftover chicken meat, 1 large salad or 1 small tub coleslaw in reduced-calorie dressing, 1 large slice bread or 2 small slices bread with little low-fat spread.

Main meal

Family Choice: 1 portion Toad in the Hole (see recipe page 280), 3 tablespoons baked beans, 3 tablespoons mashed potato.

Quick and Easy: 2 large pork or beef sausages, well grilled, 5 tablespoons instant mashed potato, 3 tablespoons baked beans, 1 diet yogurt or apple.

Heat and Serve: 1 Findus Toad in the Hole, 3 tablespoons baked beans, 3 tablespoons instant mashed potato.

Takeaway: 1 Spud U Like Spud Plus with sausage and bean filling.

DAY 2

Breakfast

EITHER 2 large slices bread with a little low-fat spread and 4 teaspoons reduced-sugar jam or marmalade, ½ grapefruit or 4 oz (115 g) canned grapefruit segments

OR 2 Weetabix or Shredded Wheat, ¼ pint (150 ml) milk, 1 small slice bread with a little low-fat spread, ½ grapefruit or 4 oz (115 g) canned grapefruit segments.

Light meal

EITHER 2 oz (55 g) Cheddar cheese, melted, on 1 large slice toast spread with a little low-fat spread, topped with 1 sliced tomato, salad garnish

OR 2 oz (55 g) Cheddar cheese with 1 large slice bread or 3 cream crackers and a little low-fat spread, 1 dessertspoon pickle of choice, salad garnish.

Main meal

Family Choice: 1 portion Corned Beef Hash (see recipe page 279), 3 tablespoons sweetcorn, 2 oz (55 g) green beans.

Quick and Easy: 4 × 1 oz (30 g) slices corned beef, 1 × 4 oz (115 g) carton Shape potato salad, large mixed salad, 1 dessertspoon pickle of choice, 1 banana.

Heat and Serve: 1 Findus Dinner Supreme Beef Madras, 1 dessertspoon chutney of choice, tomato salad.

Takeaway: 1 doner kebab.

DAY 3

Breakfast

EITHER 1 average kipper fillet, 1 medium slice bread with a little low-fat spread, 4 fl oz (120 ml) unsweetened orange, grapefruit or pineapple juice

OR 2 medium slices bread with a little low-fat spread and 2 teaspoons reduced-sugar jam or marmalade, 1 banana or diet yogurt.

Light meal

EITHER 1 × 10½ oz (300 g) can Heinz Tomato and Lentil or Pea and Ham soup, 1 medium slice bread with little low-fat spread, 1 apple

OR 3 oz (85 g) very lean ham or 2 oz (55 g) pâté of choice, 1 medium slice bread with a little low-fat spread or 2 crispbreads, tomato salad.

Main meal

Family Choice: 1 portion Spanish Omelette (see recipe page 256), 4 oz (115 g) oven chips, 4 tablespoons peas.

Quick and Easy: 2 size-3 eggs, dry-fried, 5 oz (140 g) oven chips, 4 tablespoons peas, 1 small slice bread.

Heat and Serve: 1 individual cheese and onion or mushroom quiche, large salad or 3 tablespoons sweetcorn salad, 1 large slice bread with a little low-fat spread.

Takeaway: 1 individual thin and crispy cheese and tomato pizza.

DAY 4

Breakfast

As Day 2.

Light meal

EITHER 1 × 8 oz (225 g) can baked beans in tomato or barbecue sauce on 1 medium slice toast with a little low-fat spread, 1 apple

OR 1 × 3½ oz (100 g) can tuna, well drained, 1 average bread roll or 2 small slices bread with a little low-fat spread, 1 × 4 oz (115 g) tub Shape salad, any variety except potato, salad garnish.

Main meal

Family Choice: 1 portion Lasagne (see recipe page 268), salad.

Quick and Easy: 4 oz (115 g) beefburger, well grilled or dry-fried, 5 oz (140 g) oven chips, 4 tablespoons peas or sweetcorn or baked beans, 1 dessertspoon relish of choice, 1 orange.

Heat and Serve: EITHER 1 Findus Spicy Beef and Pork Lasagne

OR 1 Findus Cannelloni, both with salad.

Takeaway: 1 regular hamburger and regular French fries.

DAY 5

Breakfast

As Day 1.

Light meal

EITHER 2 size-3 eggs, poached or scrambled with $\frac{1}{4}$ oz (7 g) butter, on 1 medium slice toast with a little low-fat spread, 1 diet yogurt

OR 1 Scotch egg with large salad, 1 teaspoon mayonnaise or dressing of choice, 1 diet yogurt.

Main meal

Family Choice: 1 portion Monkfish Kebabs (see recipe page 260), 6 tablespoons boiled rice, 1 dessertspoon chutney of choice, salad.

Quick and Easy: 4 fish fingers, grilled or dry-fried, 5 tablespoons instant mash with $\frac{1}{4}$ oz (7 g) butter or 4 oz (115 g) oven chips, 3 tablespoons peas or baked beans, 1 banana.

Heat and Serve: 1 individual cod crumble, 4 tablespoons instant mash, 3 tablespoons peas or sweetcorn.

Takeaway: Wimpy Fish and Chips.

DAY 6

Breakfast

EITHER 2 rashers lean bacon, well grilled, 4 oz (115 g) mushrooms, stir-fried, 1 medium slice bread with a little low-fat spread, 4 fl oz (120 ml) unsweetened orange, grapefruit or pineapple juice

OR 1 Weetabix or Shredded Wheat with 4 fl oz (120 ml) milk, 1 medium slice bread with a little low-fat spread and 1 teaspoon reduced-sugar jam or marmalade.

Light meal

EITHER 1 Pizza Toast (see recipe page 254)

OR 1 Findus French Bread Pizza, any variety, both with salad.

OR Ploughman's Lunch – 1½ oz (45 g) Cheddar cheese or 3 oz (85 g) reduced-fat Cheddar-style cheese, 1½ oz (45 g) French bread or 1 large slice bread with a little low-fat spread, 1 dessertspoon pickle, salad garnish.

Main meal

Family Choice: 1 portion Chicken Curry (see recipe page 263), 6 tablespoons boiled rice, 1 poppadom, 1 dessertspoon chutney of choice, 1 sliced banana or 3 tablespoons thick natural yogurt with chopped cucumber.

Quick and Easy: ½ × 15 oz (425 g) can chicken curry, 6 tablespoons boiled rice, 1 vegetable samosa or 2 grilled poppadoms, 1 dessertspoon chutney of choice.

Heat and Serve: 1 Findus Tandoori Chicken Masala, 1 dessertspoon chutney.

Takeaway: 1 portion Tandoori chicken, 1 portion rice or 1 naan or chapati.

DAY 7

Breakfast

EITHER 6 oz (170 g) smoked haddock, 1 size-3 egg, poached, ¼ oz (7 g) butter, 1 medium slice bread

OR 3 oz (85 g) crisply cooked lean bacon or ham, 4 oz (115 g) sliced mushrooms, stir-fried, or 1 dry-fried size-3 egg, 1 small slice bread.

OR as Day 1.

Light meal

EITHER 1 × 10½ oz (300 g) can cream of tomato soup, 1 average bread roll or 2 small slices bread, 1 apple

OR 1 × 3½ oz (100 g) can salmon or sardines or tuna, well drained, 1 average bread roll or 2 small slices bread, a little low-fat spread, salad.

Main meal

Family Choice: 4 oz (115 g) lean well-done roast beef, leg of lamb or pork, 6 oz (170 g) baked potato or 2 small chunks roast potato, 4 oz (115 g) greens or cauliflower or carrots, 3 tablespoons peas, 2 teaspoons mint, horseradish or apple sauce, 2 tablespoons thin gravy, 1 × 6 oz (170 g) portion apple pie or crumble with 2 tablespoons single cream.

Quick and Easy: 1 individual steak and kidney or beef and onion pie, 5 tablespoons mashed potato, 5 tablespoons mixed peas and carrots.

Heat and Serve: 1 Birds Eye Roast Beef Platter or Prizesteak Platter, 1 individual small apple pie.

Takeaway: 1 portion beef and peppers in oyster sauce, ½ portion special rice.

Sunday brunch exchange

If you prefer, have the following brunch instead of both the Day 7 breakfast and the light meal. (So you just have a brunch and main meal today.)

2 size-3 eggs, fried, 1 chipolata or 1 good slice black pudding, well fried or grilled, 1 potato cake, dry-fried or grilled, 2 back rashers, well grilled, 3 tablespoons baked beans or 2 tablespoons dry-fried mushrooms, 1 medium slice bread with a little low-fat spread, 1 dessertspoon sauce of choice.

DAY 8

Breakfast

As Day 1.

Light meal

EITHER 1 portion frozen boil-in-bag cod in butter sauce, 5 tablespoons instant mash, 4 tablespoons peas, 1 diet yogurt

OR 3 oz (85 g) leftover roast meat, lean only, or corned beef or tongue, 1 large slice bread or 2 small slices bread with a little low-fat spread, 1 small tub coleslaw in reduced-calorie dressing, salad.

Main meal

Family Choice: 1 portion Tagliatelle with Ham (see recipe page 266), salad, 1 orange or apple.

Quick and Easy: 5 oz (140 g) gammon steak, 4 oz (115 g) oven chips or 6 oz (170 g) baked potato with ¼ oz (7 g) butter, 4 tablespoons peas or broad beans.

Heat and Serve: EITHER 1 McCain Oven Meal and Chips, salad

OR 1 Birds Eye Gammon Steak Platter, salad, 1 orange or apple PLUS extra 100 calories' worth of any Extra (see pages 189–92).

Takeaway: 1 portion barbecued spare ribs, ½ portion special rice.

DAY 9

Breakfast

As Day 2.

Light meal

EITHER 5-in cheese and tomato pizza with 1 oz (30 g) extra Cheddar cheese grated on, salad

OR Ploughman's, as Day 6.

Main meal

Family Choice: EITHER 1 portion Basic Mince (see recipe page 270), 6 tablespoons mashed potato or 6 oz (170 g)

baked potato with $\frac{1}{4}$ oz (7 g) butter, 4 oz (115 g) green beans
OR 1 portion Chilli con Carne (see recipe page 271), 7 tablespoons boiled rice, salad.

Quick and Easy: EITHER 4 oz (115 g) steak grill or 2 chilli beef crispy pancakes, dry-fried, 4 oz (115 g) oven chips, 4 tablespoons peas or sweetcorn

OR $\frac{1}{2}$ can Campbell's Chilli con Carne with 6 tablespoons boiled rice, salad, 1 apple.

Heat and Serve: 1 Birds Eye Chilli con Carne with Rice, salad, 1 banana.

Takeaway: Spud U Like Spud 'n One, Chilli con Carne variety, with butter.

DAY 10

Breakfast

As Day 3.

Light meal

EITHER 1 size-3 egg, dry-fried, 4 oz (115 g) oven chips, 1 tomato

OR 1 size-3 egg, hard-boiled, 2 large slices bread with a little low-fat spread, salad and 2 teaspoons mayonnaise.

Main meal

Family Choice: 1 portion Sweet and Sour Pork (see recipe page 277), 6 tablespoons boiled rice or 5 oz (140 g) boiled noodles, salad.

Quick and Easy: 1 average trimmed pork chop, grilled, 4 croquette potatoes or 6 oz (170 g) savoury noodles, 4 tablespoons peas or 4 oz (115 g) broccoli, 1 portion Barbecue Sauce (see recipe page 252) or 2 tablespoons stuffing from packet.

Heat and Serve: 1 Mr Chang's Spare Ribs in Barbecue Sauce, 4 tablespoons boiled rice.

Takeaway: 1 portion sweet and sour pork balls with sauce and prawn crackers.

DAY 11

Breakfast

As Day 4.

Light meal

EITHER 3 fish fingers, grilled, 3 tablespoons mashed potato, 4 tablespoons peas or baked beans

OR 1 3½ oz (100 g) can tuna, sardines or salmon, well drained, 1 medium slice bread with a little low-fat spread, salad, 2 teaspoons mayonnaise.

Main meal

Family Choice: 4 pork or beef chipolata sausages, well grilled or fried, 1 size-3 egg, dry-fried, 5 oz (140 g) oven chips.

Quick and Easy: As Family Choice.

Heat and Serve: 1 Bejam or Asda Sausage and Mash, 5 tablespoons baked beans.

Takeaway: 1 individual thin and crispy pizza, any variety.

DAY 12

Breakfast

As Day 5.

Light meal

EITHER Cauliflower cheese — 10 oz (285 g) lightly cooked cauliflower topped with 1 portion Cheese Sauce (see recipe page 251) with 1 oz (30 g) extra Cheddar cheese grated over top and browned under grill, salad

OR 1½ oz (45 g) Cheddar cheese or 2 oz (55 g) Edam or Brie with 3 cream crackers or crispbreads, a little low-fat spread, 1 dessertspoon pickle of choice, 1 tomato.

Main meal

Family Choice: 1 portion Tuna Florentino (see recipe page 257), 6 oz (170 g) boiled potatoes, 5 oz (140 g) broccoli, 1 apple.

Quick and Easy: 2 fish cakes, dry-fried, or 1 oven crispy cod steak (battered), 6 oz (170 g) oven chips or potato bites, 4 tablespoons peas or sweetcorn.

Heat and Serve: 1 Birds Eye Seafood Flaky Bake, 4 tablespoons mashed potato, 4 oz (115 g) green beans.

Takeaway: 1 portion chip shop cod or haddock in batter, ½ portion chips and 1 portion mushy peas (optional).

DAY 13

Breakfast

As Day 6.

Light meal

EITHER 2 oz (55 g) beefburger, well grilled or fried, 2 croquette potatoes or 1 small bap, 4 tablespoons baked beans or 1 small tub coleslaw in reduced-calorie dressing, 1 teaspoon relish

OR 4 oz (115 g) very lean ham, 1 average bread roll with a little low-fat spread, salad, 1 teaspoon dressing of choice.

Main meal

Family Choice: EITHER 1 portion Moussaka (see recipe page 271)

OR 1 portion Beef Enchiladas (see recipe page 272), both with salad, 1 banana or 1 French-style yogurt.

Quick and Easy: 3 Mexican taco shells, cooked as instructed and filled with ½ can beef taco filling, topped with taco sauce and chopped salad items of choice, salad, 1 banana.

Heat and Serve: 1 Findus Moussaka, salad, 1 banana.
Takeaway: As Day 3 or 4.

DAY 14

Breakfast
As Day 7.

Light meal
EITHER 1 French Bread Pizza, any variety, salad
  OR 2 oz (55 g) liver pâté, 3 crispbreads or 2 small slices
bread with low-fat spread, salad, 1 apple.

Main meal
Family Choice: 4 oz (115 g) roast chicken or turkey, 3 small
chunks roast potato or 8 oz (225 g) baked potato with ¼ oz
(7 g) butter, 4 oz (115 g) mixed peas and carrots, 4 oz (115 g)
broccoli or sprouts, 2 tablespoons thin gravy, 2 tablespoons packet stuffing.
Quick and Easy: 1 average roast chicken or Tandoori
chicken portion, 5 tablespoons instant mash or 6 oz (170 g)
baked potato with ¼ oz (7 g) butter or 5 oz (140 g) oven
chips or 2 medium slices bread with a little low-fat spread,
3 tablespoons peas or sweetcorn, salad.
Heat and Serve: 1 Birds Eye Roast Chicken Platter, 1
banana or diet yogurt.
Takeaway: EITHER 1 Kentucky Fried Chicken Dinner for
One with beans and chips
  OR 6 chicken McNuggets with regular French fries
(McDonald's).

Sunday brunch exchange
As Day 7.

8 · THE JUNK FOOD DIET – 3

· THE PICK YOUR OWN PLAN ·

Now you're ready to pick your own Junk Food Diet – and it's simplicity itself, with the help of the meal listings that follow. All you have to do is pick meals and extras to your own dieting calorie total – 1,000, 1,250 or 1,500.

To help you, here is a breakdown of the calorie-counted meal categories available for you to choose from. The detailed contents of these categories are given on pages 142–94.

Breakfasts and snacks, cold	200, 250, 300
Breakfasts and snacks, hot	200, 250, 300
Light meals, cold	250, 300, 400
Light meals, brunches and suppers, hot	300, 400, 500
Toast meals	250, 300, 400
Bread and sandwich meals	250, 300, 400
Potato meals	250, 400
Main meals, family choice	300, 400, 500, 600
Main meals, quick and easy	300, 400, 500, 600
Main meals, heat and serve	300, 400, 500, 600
Top takeaways	300, 400, 500, 600, 700, 800, 900
Vegetables, pasta and rice	25, 50, 75, 100, 150
Fruit and juices	25, 50, 75, 100
Milk and yoghurt	50, 75, 100
Treats, snacks and extras	25, 50, 75, 100, 150, 200, 300

The only things to remember – apart from the rules listed in Chapter 6, which still apply here, are:

· Have no more than one meal from any one meal section a day, and get as much variety into your daily diet as you can. For instance, if you had an egg meal for breakfast, don't have egg for lunch and supper as well.

· Some vegetables are included within many meals. You should also use the vegetables on the Unlimited lists as much as you like, and if you want extra vegetables, there are plenty to choose from within the listings.

· Try to get a daily portion of milk or yogurt and fruit, like you did on the Set Diet.

· Your daily maximum Treats/Extras allowance is still 100 calories if you're on 1,000 calories a day, 200 calories if you're on 1,250 calories a day and 300 if you're on 1,500 calories a day. But if you prefer not to use these calories on treats you can, of course, use them on other foods listed.

· Try to have several meals/snacks a day rather than just one big meal. If you're on 1,000 calories a day, the maximum calorie count for any one meal should be 500. If you're on 1,250 or 1,500 the maximum should be 600. The only exception to this rule is that if you're on 1,250 you can have an occasional takeaway of 700, and if you're on 1,500 you can have an occasional takeaway of up to 900. But on those 'high takeaway' days, you would be wise to forgo your day's Treats allowance and spend the calories on something else, such as a fruit and yogurt snack or a small meal.

Don't forget, you can return to the Set Diet any time you like, and you should move *down* a calorie band if your weight loss slows right down or stops.

As to brand names, when I haven't specified one before a product, any brand will do: for instance, fish fingers, fish cakes and instant mash vary by hardly any calories from brand to brand. But sometimes calories do vary widely, so when I've specified brand names it's best to stick to them, which is why I've used only widely available brands or top supermarket labels.

Before you start, take a good look through the listings to familiarize yourself with them. Spend a while planning out some combinations that appeal to you and working out meal patterns that are compatible with the way you live.

· EXAMPLES ·

Here are two examples of how you might plan out a day's menu from the lists, according to your own needs.

Tina is on 1,250 calories a day. She is at work and needs a quick breakfast, a packed lunch and a very quick family evening meal during the week. She chooses:

Cold breakfast – 200 calories
Cold lunch – 300 calories
Fruit – 50 calories
Quick and easy main meal – 400 calories
Dessert from Treats list – 100 calories
Extra butter from Extras list – 100 calories
Milk for use in drinks – 100 calories

However, on a Sunday she prefers a late morning brunch and a main roast meal with dessert in the evening, and so she chooses:

Brunch – 400 calories
Sandwich meal – 250 calories
Main meal – 300 calories
Dessert (from Treats list) – 200 calories
Fruit – 50 calories
Milk – 50 calories

Emma, a teenager on 1,500 calories, likes to snack during

the day, and this Saturday wants to look forward to a takeaway tuck-in with her friends. This is what she chooses:

Cold breakfast – 200 calories
Early lunch of a sandwich meal – 250 calories
Fruit – 50 calories
Early tea of a toast meal – 250 calories
Diet yogurt – 50 calories
Takeaway supper – 700 calories

She prefers not to use her 300 calorie Treats allowance, having her takeaway meal and a breakfast instead.

Plan out your own meals this way, and you'll find losing weight a pleasure.

Please note: When using the listings that follow, you should pick one item from the first column and then stay within that horizontal ruled section when picking the rest of your meal from columns two and three.

Breakfasts and snacks, cold – 200 calories

Pick one of these	Plus	
Pick one of these 2 Shredded Wheat 1½ oz (45 g) muesli 1½ oz (45 g) grapenuts 2 Weetabix + 1 teaspoon sugar	*Plus* ¼ pint (150 ml) skimmed milk	
Pick one of these 1 oz (30 g) Cornflakes 1 oz (30 g) Frosties 1 oz (30 g) Fruit 'n' Fibre 1 oz (30 g) Raisin Splitz 1 oz (30 g) Shreddies 1 oz (30 g) Special K 1 oz (30 g) Start 1 oz (30 g) Sugar Puffs 1 oz (30 g) Weetaflakes	*Plus one of these* ¼ pint (150 ml) skimmed milk 4 fl oz (120 ml) semi-skimmed milk	*Plus one of these* Any 1 portion from 50-calorie fruit selection on page 187 ¼ pint (150 ml) unsweetened orange, grapefruit or pineapple juice
1 oz (30 g) All Bran 1 oz (30 g) Bran Buds 1 oz (30 g) Bran Flakes	¼ pint (150 ml) skimmed milk 4 fl oz (120 ml) semi-skimmed milk	1 banana 1 thin slice bread with a little low- fat spread, plain or with Marmite
1 Nouvelle or Ski or Prize fruit yogurt	1 banana	
1 Thick and Creamy yogurt 1 Greek-style yogurt	½ grapefruit 1 teaspoon honey	

1 medium-cut slice bread from a large loaf with a little low-fat spread 3 crispbreads with a little low-fat spread 2 slices Hi-Bran bread from a small loaf with a little low-fat spread	3 teaspoons honey 3 teaspoons marmalade 3 teaspoons jam 6 teaspoons reduced-sugar jam 1 oz (30 g) medium-fat soft cheese 1 oz (30 g) cheese spread 1 oz (30 g) lean ham 1 oz (30 g) chicken 1 oz (30 g) lite pâté	1 diet yogurt Any 1 portion from 50-calorie fruit selection on page 187 1 Shape Fromage Frais
2 slices bread from a medium-cut loaf with a little low-fat spread.		
2 slices bread from a thin-cut loaf with a little low-fat spread 1 wholemeal scone with a little low-fat spread 1 currant bun with a little low-fat spread	3 teaspoons jam 3 teaspoons marmalade 6 teaspoons reduced-sugar jam 6 teaspoons reduced-sugar marmalade 1 portion from 50-calorie fruit selection on page 187	

Breakfasts and snacks, cold – 250 calories

Pick one of these 1 Thick and Creamy yogurt 1 Greek-style yogurt	Plus one of these 1 banana	Plus one of these 1 slice bread from a thin-cut loaf with a little low-fat spread

1½ oz (45 g) muesli 2 slices bread from thin-cut loaf with a little low-fat spread	¼ pint (150 ml) skimmed milk 1 diet yoghurt	1 portion from any 50-calorie fruit selection on page 187 1 slice Hi-Bran bread from a small loaf with a little low-fat spread
1 oz (30 g) Cornflakes 1 oz (30 g) Frosties 1 oz (30 g) Fruit 'n Fibre 1 oz (30 g) Raisin Splitz 1 oz (30 g) Shreddies 1 oz (30 g) Special K 1 oz (30 g) Start 1 oz (30 g) Sugar Puffs 1 oz (30 g) Weetaflakes	¼ pint (150 ml) skimmed milk 4 fl oz (120 ml) semi-skimmed milk	1 slice bread from a thin-cut loaf with a little low-fat spread and 1 teaspoon jam or marmalade
1 average bread roll with a little low-fat spread	1 oz (30 g) Cheddar cheese	
2 slices bread from a thin cut loaf with a little low-fat spread	1 diet yogurt 6 teaspoons reduced-sugar jam 6 teaspoons reduced-sugar marmalade 1 oz (25 g) cheese spread 1 oz (25 g) medium-fat soft cheese	
2 slices bread from a thin cut loaf with a little low-fat spread	1 large banana 2 oz (55 g) lean ham 1 French-style yogurt	

Breakfasts and snacks, cold — 300 calories

Pick one of these	Plus one of these	Plus one of these
1 oz (30 g) Cornflakes 1 oz (30 g) Frosties 1 oz (30 g) Fruit 'n Fibre 1 oz (30 g) Raisin Splitz 1 oz (30 g) Shreddies 1 oz (30 g) Special K 1 oz (30 g) Start 1 oz (30 g) Sugar Puffs 1 oz (30 g) Weetaflakes	¼ pint (150 ml) skimmed milk 4 fl oz (120 ml) semi-skimmed milk	1 slice bread from medium-cut loaf with a little butter and reduced-sugar jam plus 4 fl oz (120 ml) fruit juice
2 oz (55 g) muesli	¼ pint (150 ml) skimmed milk	Any 1 portion from 50-calorie fruit selection on page 187 ¼ pint (150 ml) unsweetened fruit juice
2 Shredded wheat	¼ pint (150 ml) skimmed milk 4 fl oz (120 ml) semi-skimmed milk	1 large banana 1 slice bread from medium-cut loaf with a little low-fat spread and 1 teaspoon jam or marmalade
2 slices bread from a medium-cut loaf with a little low-fat spread	1 oz (30 g) Cheddar cheese 2 slices lean ham and 1 teaspoon pickle	

145

Breakfasts and snacks, hot – 200 calories

Pick one of these	Plus one of these	Plus one of these
1 size-3 egg, poached 1 size-3 egg, boiled	2 rashers streaky bacon, well grilled 1 large rasher back bacon, well grilled	2 tomatoes, raw or grilled
4 oz (115 g) baked beans 4 oz (115 g) mushrooms, dry-fried in ¼ oz (7 g) butter	1 large rasher back bacon, well grilled 2 chipolatas, well grilled 1 large low-fat sausage, grilled 1 slice bread from a medium-cut loaf with a little low-fat spread	¼ grapefruit
1 oz (30 g) porridge oats 1 oz (30 g) Ready Brek 1 oz (30 g) Warm Start	¼ pint (150 ml) skimmed milk, water as necessary	2 teaspoons sugar, syrup or honey
5 oz (140 g) baked beans	1 slice bread from a medium-cut loaf with a little low-fat spread	

Breakfasts and snacks, hot – 250 calories

Pick one of these	Plus one of these	Plus one of these
1½ oz (45 g) porridge oats	¼ pint (150 ml) skimmed milk, water as necessary	2 teaspoons sugar, syrup or honey
1 size-3 egg, poached	2 oz (55 g) lean ham 2 rashers streaky bacon 2 chipolatas, well grilled 5 oz (140 g) baked beans	1 slice bread from a thin cut loaf with a little low-fat spread

1 size-3 egg, fried 4 oz (115 g) mushrooms, dry-fried in ¼ oz (7 g) butter	1 medium back rasher, well grilled	1 slice bread from a thin-cut loaf with a little low-fat spread
1 × 3½ (100 g) can soft herring roes	1 slice bread from a thin-cut loaf with a little low-fat spread	
1 size-3 egg, fried	2 medium back rashers, well grilled	1 crispbread with low-fat spread ½ grapefruit 2 oz (55 g) mushrooms, grilled

Breakfasts and snacks, hot – 300 calories

Pick one of these 1 × 7 oz (200 g) pack buttered smoked haddock	Plus one of these 1 slice bread from a medium-cut loaf with a little low-fat spread 1 slice bread from a thin-cut loaf with a little low-fat spread, ½ grapefruit	Plus one of these
1 size-3 egg, fried 2 size-3 eggs, poached	1 medium back rasher, well grilled 1 large pork sausage, grilled 2 rashers streaky bacon, well grilled 2 chipolatas, well grilled	1 slice bread from a medium-cut loaf with a little low-fat spread 2 slices Melba toast or rye crispbread with a little low-fat spread

Light meals, cold – 250 calories

Pick one of these	Plus one of these	Plus one of these
2 cold well-grilled chipolatas	4 oz (115 g) cold boiled potato	1 dessertspoon pickle of choice
3 oz (85 g) very lean ham	2-in slice French bread	1 dessertspoon made-up packet stuffing
3½ oz (100 g) chicken meat or chicken roll	1 slice bread from a medium-cut loaf with a little butter	1 teaspoon mayonnaise
4 small slices garlic sausage (2 oz, 55 g)	3 crispbreads with low-fat spread	2 teaspoons mustard
2 oz (55 g) corned beef	1 × 3½ oz (100 g) tub Shape coleslaw or Shape potato salad + 1	
Generous 1 oz (30 g) Cheddar	slice Hi-Bran bread from a small loaf	
2 oz (55 g) reduced-fat Cheddar	2 cream crackers with little butter	
1½ oz (45 g) Edam or Brie or Danish Blue		
2 size-4 egg, hard boiled		
1 × 3½ oz (105 g) can pink salmon		
1 × 3½ oz (100 g) can tuna, well drained		
3 oz (85 g) lite pâté		
2 oz (55 g) standard liver pâté		
2 oz (55 g) tongue		
3½ oz (100 g) turkey		
3 oz (85 g) lean roast beef		

Light meals, cold – 300 calories

Pick one of these	Plus one of these
1 Scotch egg	Salad from Unlimited list
Egg mayonnaise—three size-3 hard-boiled egg halves plus two level tablespoons reduced-calorie mayonnaise	2-in slice French bread
	2 slices Hi-Bran bread from a small loaf with a little low-fat spread
1 large cold cooked chicken portion	1 × 4 oz (115 g) Shape Curried Potato Salad
4 oz (115 g) hummus	3 oz (85 g) rice salad
2 tablespoons taramasalata	3 oz (85 g) sweetcorn salad
1 × 4 oz (115 g) slice quiche	1 × 3½ oz (100 g) tub reduced-calorie coleslaw
3 oz (85 g) corned beef	1 slice bread from medium-cut loaf with butter
1½ oz (45 g) Cheddar	1 mini pitta
2 oz (55 g) Danish Blue	3 crispbreads with low-fat spread
1 × 3½ oz (100 g) can red salmon	
1 × 4½ oz (120 g) can sardines, well drained	
2½ oz (70 g) standard pâté	
3 oz (85 g) liver sausage	
1 × 6½ oz (185 g) can John West Tuna in Mayonnaise	
1 × 6½ oz (185 g) can John West Tuna in Tomato sauce	

1 × 2½ oz (70 g) (party) pork pie 1 large 3½ oz (100 g) sausage roll 1 Kraft Cheese and Onion Pastry	Salad from Unlimited list + 1 teaspoon mayonnaise

Light meals, cold – 400 calories

Pick one of these	Plus one of these Salad from Unlimited list	Plus one of these
1 Cornish pasty 1 individual Walls or Kraft Chicken, Chicken and Vegetable or Chicken and Mushroom Pie 1 individual cheese and onion quiche		
2 oz (55 g) Cheddar	2-in slice French bread	2 dessertspoons pickle 2 teaspoons low-fat spread
2 oz (55 g) reduced-fat Cheddar	3-in slice French bread	2 dessertspoons pickle 2 teaspoons low-fat spread
½ × 6½ oz (185 g) can John West Tuna and Sweetcorn in Mayonnaise	1 pitta bread	Chopped salad
½ × 6½ oz (185 g) can John West Tuna in Curry Sauce	1 pitta bread	Chopped salad + 1 banana
1 portion Paradise Chicken (see recipe page 265)	5 tablespoons cold cooked rice tossed in oil-free dressing	

Light meals, brunches and suppers, hot – 300 calories

Pick one of these	Plus one of these	Plus one of these
	1 mini pitta 1 slice bread from thin-cut loaf with a little low-fat spread	
3 fish fingers, grilled	4 oz (115 g) boiled potato	Any portion from 50-calorie fruit selection on page 187
2 fish cakes, grilled	3 oz (85 g) boiled rice	3 tablespoons sweetcorn
1 × 5 oz (140 g) breaded plaice fillet, grilled or ovenbaked	1 slice bread from medium-cut loaf with butter	3 tablespoons peas
1 portion boil-in-bag cod in butter sauce	2 oz (55 g) oven chips	3 tablespoons baked beans
1 small chicken breast portion, baked or grilled plain or with Tandoori or Chinese-style coating	1 size-3 egg, dry-fried	
4 Asda chicken fingers, baked	2 croquette potatoes	
1 Matthews Golden Drummer		
1 Findus Grillado, Chilli or Plain		
3 chipolatas, well grilled or dry-fried		
3½ oz (100 g) bacon steak		
1 Padley's Chick'n Quick Chicken Breast Steak, baked		
1 Birds Eye or Findus Battered Cod Steak	1 size-3 egg, dry-fried 2 oz (55 g) oven chips	

2 large (1¼ oz, 35 g) lean back rashers, well grilled or dry-fried 1 Matthews Crisp Crumb Turkey steak, baked 1 Buxted Chicken and Sweetcorn Panbake, baked 1 Birds Eye Prizesteak, grilled 1 portion Piperade (see recipe page 255)	4 oz (115 g) instant mash 1 slice bread from a medium-cut loaf with butter	Any portion from 50-calorie fruit selection on page 187 1 diet yogurt
10 fl oz (½ pint, 300 ml) any one of these soups: Cream of Celery Chicken Mushroom Oxtail Golden Vegetable Lentil Pea and Ham	1 average bread roll 2-in slice French bread	
1 Heinz Weightwatchers Chicken in Supreme Sauce with Vegetables 1 Birds Eye Chicken and Seafood Paella 1 Chicken Tetrazzini (see recipe page 262) 1 Ross Chinese or Indian Chicken Stir-Fry		

Pick one of these	Plus one of these	Plus one of these
1 size-3 egg, dry-fried	4 oz (115 g) oven chips	

Light meals, brunches and suppers, hot – 400 calories

Pick one of these	Plus one of these	Plus one of these
Spanish Omelette (see recipe page 256)	2 oz (55 g) oven chips 1 slice bread from medium-cut loaf with butter	
1 portion Chicken Tetrazzini (see recipe page 262)	4 oz (115 g) boiled potatoes	
1 Ross Chinese Chicken or Indian Chicken Stir-Fry with added 2 oz (55 g) chicken meat or 3 oz (85 g) peeled prawns or 1 large egg 1 McCain Potato Stir-Fry, Country Beef variety		
1 portion Bejam or Birds Eye Cauliflower Cheese 1 individual quiche		
1 size-3 egg, dry-fried	2 chipolata sausages, well grilled or dry-fried	4 oz (115 g) oven chips
1 Quarterpounder beefburger	1 burger bap	Salad + 1 dessertspoon relish of choice
2 size-3 eggs, dry-fried 4 fish fingers, grilled	4 oz (115 g) oven chips	

1 portion Chicken Tikka (see recipe page 262)	6 oz (170 g) boiled rice 1 pitta plus 1 dessertspoon chutney
1 portion Risotto (see recipe page 269)	Any 1 portion from 50-calorie fruit selection on page 187
1 portion Saucy baked Eggs (see recipe page 254)	3 tablespoons instant mash 4 oz (115 g) green beans or broccoli
1 portion Egg and Potato Pie (see recipe page 256) 1 portion Macaroni Cheese (see recipe page 265)	
1 × 7½ oz (210 g) can macaroni cheese	1 slice bread from medium-cut loaf with butter
	1 banana 1 diet yoghurt

Brunches – 500 calories

Choose one of the following brunches

1 size-3 egg, dry-fried

1 lean rasher back bacon, grilled or dry-fried

2 chipolatas, well grilled or dry-fried or 2 oz (55 g, 2 small slices) black pudding

2 potato cakes or hash browns, dry-fried, baked or grilled

1 slice bread from a medium-cut loaf with low-fat spread or 1 extra egg

1 dessertspoon sauce of choice

1 potato waffle
2 slices lean back bacon, well grilled or dry-fried
2 size-3 eggs, dry-fried
2 oz (55 g) fried mushrooms or 1 thin slice bread from a small loaf

1 × 3 oz (85 g) cooked potato, sliced, sautéed and drained
2 size-3 eggs, dry-fried
2 lean rashers back bacon, well grilled or dry-fried

2 chipolatas, well grilled or dry-fried
1 size-3 egg, dry-fried
2 rashers back bacon, well grilled or dry-fried
3 tablespoons baked beans
1 slice bread from a medium-cut loaf with low-fat spread

Toast meals - 250 calories

Pick one of these	Plus
2 size-3 eggs, poached	1 slice bread from a medium-cut loaf, toasted, with a little low-fat spread
1 × 3½ oz (100 g) pack Princes Barbecued Chicken Toastie	
1 × 4½ oz (125 g) can Turkey and Ham Toast Topper	
½ × 7 oz can Chunky Chicken Supreme or Chunky Chicken Spanish Style	

2 oz (55 g) reduced-fat Cheddar, melted

4 oz (115 g) soft herring roes cooked in ¼ oz (7 g) butter

1 × 7½ oz (210 g) can spaghetti in tomato sauce

2 oz (55 g) lite Brussels pâté

2 oz (55 g) kipper spreading pâté

1 × 7½ oz (210 g) can ravioli in tomato sauce

1 × 7½ oz (210 g) can baked beans in tomato sauce or barbecue sauce

Toast meals – 300 calories

Plus
1 slice bread from a medium-cut loaf, toasted, with a little low-fat spread

Pick one of these

1 × 8 oz (225 g) can curried beans with sultanas

2 size-3 eggs, scrambled with 2 fl oz (60 ml) skimmed milk and 2 teaspoons low-fat spread

2 oz (55 g) Cheshire or Edam cheese

1 × 4½ oz (125 g) can Ham and Cheese or Mushroom and Bacon Toast Topper

4 × 2 oz (55 g) lamb's kidneys,
quartered and stir-fried in a little
low-fat spread

6 oz (170 g) mushrooms, stir-fried in
½ oz (15 g) butter

1 × 4½ oz (120 g) can sardines in oil,
well drained

1 portion Piperade (see recipe page
255)

1 Pizza Toast (see recipe page 254)

Toast meals – 400 calories

Pick one of these	Plus
1 × 8 oz (225 g) can baked beans with pork sausages or burger bites	1 slice bread from a thick-cut loaf, toasted, with a little low-fat spread
1 × 4½ oz (120 g) can sardines in tomato sauce	
1 × 7 oz (206 g) can Chunky Chicken Indian style	
1 × 7½ oz (210 g) can macaroni cheese	1 slice bread from a thick-cut loaf, toasted, with a little low-fat spread
	Any 1 portion from a 50 calorie fruit selection on page 187

Bread and sandwich meals – 250 calories

Pick one of these	Plus
1 size-3 egg, hard boiled, + 2 teaspoons reduced-calorie mayonnaise or 1 dessertspoon pickle	2 slices bread from a thin-cut loaf with a little low-fat spread
2 oz (55 g) lite pâté	
2 oz (55 g) very lean ham + 2 dessertspoons reduced-calorie coleslaw or pickle	
2½ oz (70 g) chicken or turkey roll	
2 oz (55 g) lean roast beef or pork	
1 × 3½ oz (100 g) can tuna in brine, drained	
1 × 3½ oz (100 g) can prawns, drained, plus 2 teaspoons reduced-calorie mayonnaise	
2 oz (55 g) medium-fat soft cheese	
1 good dessertspoon peanut butter	
1 Kraft Single and 1 oz (30 g) lean ham	
1 oz (30 g) Bel Paese cheese	
1 oz (30 g) Edam and 1 dessertspoon pickle	
1½ oz (40 g) reduced-fat Cheddar	
1 × 5-in Pizza	

| 1 McVitie's Pizza Slice | Any 1 portion from 50-calorie fruit selection on page 187 |
| 1 × 4½ oz (125 g) can Chicken and Mushroom Toast Toppers, warmed | 1 pitta bread |

Bread and sandwich meals – 300 calories

Pick one of these	*Plus one of these*
2 oz (55 g) pâté	2 slices bread from a thin-cut loaf with a little low-fat spread
1¼ oz (35 g) Cheddar	1 average roll with a little low-fat spread
2 oz (55 g) reduced-fat Cheddar + 1 teaspoon pickle	
1 oz (30 g) Cheddar + 1 dessertspoon pickle	
2 oz (55 g) corned beef + 1 teaspoon pickle	
2 oz (55 g) tongue	
1 × 3½ oz (105 g) can pink salmon	
3 oz (85 g) chicken meat + 1 dessertspoon reduced-calorie mayonnaise with ½ teaspoon curry powder (optional)	
1 Pizza Toast (see recipe page 254)	
1 Findus French Bread Pizza, Cheese, Bacon, Pepper and Mushroom, or Sausage, Courgette,	

Pepper and Sweetcorn variety
1 Birds Eye French Bread Pizza, Cheese and Tomato or Sausage variety
2 Sainsbury's Party Pizza Wedges

Bread and sandwich meals – 400 calories

Pick one of these	Plus
1 Asda Calzone, any variety	1 apple
½ × any 14 oz (400 g) pizza	
1 Chicken and Mushroom Pitta (see recipe page 253)	1 apple
1 Tuna Pitta (see recipe page 253)	1 apple
1 pitta filled with ½ × 6½ oz (185 g) can John West Tuna with Sweetcorn in Mayonnaise	

Potato meals – 250 calories

Pick one of these	Plus one of these	Plus
6 oz (170 g) instant mashed potato	1 size-3 egg, poached	¼ oz (7 g) butter
2 hash browns	3 tablespoons baked beans	
1 potato pancake	2 oz (55 g) medium-fat soft cheese	

6 oz (170 g) baked potato	1 slice lean back bacon, well grilled and chopped	
	Potato meals – 400 calories	
Pick one of these 8 oz (225 g) baked potato	*Plus one of these* 1¼ oz (35 g) grated Cheddar 3 tablespoons baked beans + 1 crisp lean back rasher, chopped 2 oz (55 g) very lean ham, chopped 1 large poached egg 1 × 4¼ oz (125 g) portion John West Tuna in Curry Sauce 1 × 4¼ oz (125 g) portion John West Tuna in Barbecue Sauce	*Plus* ¼ oz (7 g) butter ½ oz (15 g) butter
1 McCain Potato Stir-Fry, Country Beef variety 1 Egg and Potato Pie (see recipe page 256)	4 oz (115 g) green beans	
8 oz (225 g) baked potato	4 oz (115 g) stir-fried mushrooms using ½ oz (15 g) butter	
2 Birds Eye Jacket Potato Halves with Bacon and Cheese or Cheese and Onion		

Main meals, family choice – 300 calories

Pick one of these	Plus one of these	Plus
1 portion Basic Mince (see recipe page 270)	4 oz (115 g) boiled potato	Vegetables or salad of choice from unlimited list
1 portion Beef Stir-Fry (see recipe page 274)	4 oz (115 g) baked potato	
1 portion Turkey Kebabs (see recipe page 264)	5 oz (140 g) instant mash	
	5 tablespoons boiled rice	
1 portion Chicken Tikka (see recipe page 262)	3 oz (85 g) boiled noodles	
	¼ pack Golden or Mushroom Savoury Rice	
1 portion Scampi Provençale (see recipe page 259)	2 croquette potatoes, baked or grilled	
1 portion Cod Creole (see recipe page 259)	1 medium chunk roast potato	
½ × 15 oz (425 g) can Campbell's Beef Curry	2 oz (55 g) oven chips	
¼ of a fish casserole made with 1½ lb (675 g) white fish fillet + 1 carton Knorr Tomato and Onion Recipe Sauce		
½ × 8 oz (225 g) pack Tesco Italian-style chicken bites, baked		

½ × 1 lb (450 g) pack Asda Chicken Italienne

4 oz (115 g) lean roast beef, leg of lamb or pork with 2 tablespoons thin gravy

5 oz (140 g) roast chicken or 4 oz (115 g) roast chicken + 1 tablespoon stuffing

½ × 15 oz (425 g) can Chesswood Curry with Chicken and Mushrooms

½ + 1¼ lb (570 g) pack St Michael Seafood Pasta

½ × 1⅛ lb (510 g) pack St Michael Tagliatelle

Main meals, family choice – 400 calories

Pick one of these	Plus one of these	Plus
4 oz (115 g) well-roast shoulder of lamb or duck, including crisp skin	6 oz (170 g) baked potato	Any vegetable or salad item from unlimited list
1 portion Chicken Curry (see recipe page 263)	6 tablespoons boiled rice + 1 dessertspoon chutney of choice	
1 portion Lamb Kebabs (see recipe page 277)	5 oz (140 g) boiled noodles	
½ × 1 lb (450 g) pack or tin chilli con carne (not including rice)	5 oz (140 g) potato, mashed with skimmed milk and low-fat spread	
	2 small chunks roast potato	
	3 oz (85 g) oven chips	

5 oz (140 g) lean gammon from boiled or roast joint	4 oz (115 g) instant mash + plus 3 tablespoons peas or broad beans or 4 oz (115 g) green beans	Any vegetable or salad item from unlimited list
½ × 12 oz (340 g) pack Safeway Sweet and Sour Diced Pork		
½ × 15 oz (425 g) can Campbell's Chicken Curry		
½ × 1 lb (450 g) pack Buxted Chicken Crunchies, baked		
½ × 1⅛ lb (510 g) pack Tesco Chicken Chasseur		
½ × 12 oz (325 g) pack Tesco Beef Stroganoff		
¼ × 1 lb (450 g) Sainsbury's Savoury Pie with Beef and Vegetables		
½ × 1 lb (450 g) Asda Crofter's Pie		
½ × 1 lb (450 g) Safeway or Tesco Hot Pot		
1 portion Fisherman's Pie (see recipe page 258)	4 oz (115 g) boiled potato	
1 portion Chicken Tetrazzini (see recipe page 262)	4 oz (115 g) baked potato	
1 portion Spanish Omelette (see recipe page 256)	5 oz (140 g) instant mash	
1 portion Chilli con Carne (see recipe page 271)	5 tablespoons boiled rice	
	3 oz (85 g) boiled noodles	
	¼ pack Golden or Mushroom Savoury Rice	

1 portion Beef Goulash (see recipe page 273)	2 croquette potatoes, baked or grilled
1 portion Cottage Pie (see recipe page 272)	1 medium chunk roast potato
1 portion Beef Stroganoff (see recipe page 274)	2 oz (55 g) oven chips
1 portion Boston Baked Beans (see recipe page 280)	4 oz (115 g) instant mash + 3 oz (85 g) green beans
¼ × 1 lb (450 g) Minced Beef and Onion Pie (Asda, Robirch, Tesco, Waitrose)	
¼ × 1 lb (450 g) Safeway frozen Steak and Kidney Pie	
½ × 14 oz (400 g) Tesco Cumberland Pie	
½ × 1 lb (450 g) Tesco Beef Stew and Dumplings	
½ × 15 oz (425 g) can St Michael Mild Chicken Curry	
½ × 8 oz (225 g) pack Tesco Breaded Chicken Goujons	
½ × 12 oz (340 g) pack Sainsbury's Chicken Tikka Masala	

¾ × beef curry casserole made with 1 lb (450 g) extra lean braising steak and 1 pack Knorr Recipe Curry sauce ¾ × 1 lb (450 g) Sainsbury's Chicken Plate Pie	Any 1 portion from 50-calorie fruit selection on page 187
½ × 1 lb (450 g) pack Waitrose, Sainsbury's or St Michael Moussaka 1 portion Risotto (see recipe page 269) ¼ × 1¼ lb (560 g) St Michael Cannelloni ½ × 1¼ lb (550 g) Asda Lasagne Verdi ½ × 1½ lb (510 g) Sainsbury's Lasagne Verdi	

Main meals, family choice – 500 calories

Pick one of these	Plus one of these	Plus one of these
1 portion Beef Curry (see recipe page 275)	6 oz (170 g) baked potato	
1 portion Sweet and Sour Pork (see recipe page 277)	6 tablespoons boiled rice + 1 dessertspoon chutney of choice	
1 portion Liver Paprika (see recipe page 278)	5 oz (140 g) boiled noodles	
1 portion Tuna Florentino (see recipe page 257)	5 oz (140 g) potato, mashed with skimmed milk and low-fat spread 2 small chunks roast potato	

½ × 1 lb (450 g) pack St Michael Beef Stew

½ × 17 oz (482 g) pack Asda or Safeway Beef Stew with Dumplings

¼ × Sainsbury's Deep-filled Chicken and Ham Pie or Steak and Kidney Pie

¼ × St Michael 1 lb (450 g) Plate Pie, any variety

⅓ × 12½ oz (345 g) Sainsbury's Baked Mince Roll

½ × 14 oz (400 g) pack Asda Chicken Supreme

½ × 1 lb (450 g) pack St Michael Fish Crumble

1 portion Corned Beef Hash (see recipe page 279)

1 portion Toad in the Hole (see recipe page 280)

½ × 1 lb (450 g) pack St Michael Chicken Italienne

¼ × 15 oz (425 g) Sainsbury's Minced Beef and Onion Pie

½ × 1 lb (450 g) pack Waitrose, Safeway or Tesco Pork Spare Ribs in BBQ Sauce

---

4 oz (115 g) baked beans

4 oz (115 g) peas

4 oz (115 g) sweetcorn

4 oz (115 g) broccoli or green beans + any 1 portion from 50-calorie fruit selection on page 187

5 tablespoons boiled rice

5 tablespoons instant mash

1 portion Chicken Curry (see recipe page 263)	6 tablespoons boiled rice + 1 dessertspoon chutney	1 poppadom
1 portion Beef Enchiladas (see recipe page 272)	Any 1 portion from 50-calorie fruit selection on page 187	
1 portion Moussaka (see recipe page 271)		
1 portion Tagliatelle with Ham (see recipe page 266)		
1 portion Pasta Shells with Tuna (see recipe page 267)		
1 portion Spaghetti Bolognese (see recipe page 267)		
½ × Findus Tarte à l'Oignon		

Main meals, family choice— 600 calories

Pick one of these	Plus one of these	Plus one of these
¼ × family Tiffany Steak and Mushroom Pie	4 oz (115 g) boiled potato	3 tablespoons baked beans
½ × 10½ oz (300 g) Tesco Puff Pastry Chicken and Mushroom Pie	2 oz (55 g) oven chips	3 tablespoons peas
1 portion Moussaka (see recipe page 271)	4 oz (115 g) instant mash	3 tablespoons sweetcorn
½ × 1 lb (450 g) pack Sainsbury's Moussaka		
Lasagne (see recipe page 268)	Any 1 portion from 50-calorie fruit selection on page 187	

1 portion Toad in the Hole (see recipe page 280)	6 oz (170 g) baked potato	5 oz (140 g) green beans
¼ × 19 oz (540 g) St Michael Steak and Kidney Rich Pastry Pie	6 tablespoons boiled rice + 1 dessertspoon chutney of choice	3 tablespoons peas
½ × 13 oz (375 g) St Michael Chicken Tikka Masala	6 oz (170 g) instant mash	Tomato and onion salad
½ × 18 oz (500 g) Waitrose Tandoori Chicken Masala		small tub natural yogurt with chopped cucumber
1 portion Beef Curry (see recipe page 275)	6 oz (170 g) boiled rice + 1 dessertspoon chutney of choice	1 poppadom
1 portion Sweet and Sour Pork (see recipe page 277)		4 oz (115 g) green beans
1 portion Liver Paprika (see recipe page 278)		Any 1 portion from 50-calorie fruit selection on page 187

Main meals, quick and easy – 300 calories

Pick one of these	*Plus one of these*	*Plus one of these*
2 oz (55 g) beefburger, well grilled or dry-fried	1½ oz (45 g) dry weight spaghetti, boiled	1 dessertspoon Parmesan
2 chipolatas, well grilled or dry-fried	5 oz (140 g) instant mash with ¼ oz (7 g) butter	1 dessertspoon relish
1 × 4 oz (115 g) pack Birds Eye or Sainsbury's Roast Beef and Gravy + 2 teaspoons horseradish sauce	6 oz (170 g) boiled potato	2 tablespoons baked beans
2 fish cakes, dry-fried	4 oz (115 g) boiled potato, mashed with 2 fl oz (60 ml) skimmed milk and ¼ oz (7 g) low-fat spread	2 tablespoons peas
		2 tablespoons sweetcorn

1 size-3 egg, fried 6 oz (170 g) grilled, baked or poached white fish fillet 3½ oz (100 g) round bacon steak, grilled ½ × 10½ (300 g) can Campbell's Bolognese sauce	5 oz (140 g) boiled rice 3 oz (85 g) oven chips 2 × 2 oz (55 g) chunks roast potato 1 burger bap	3 tablespoons baked beans 3 tablespoons peas 3 tablespoons sweetcorn 4 tablespoons broad beans
1 pack Birds Eye Minced Beef and Vegetables in Gravy 1 Bejam Goldenbake Turkey Steak 3 chipolatas, well grilled or dry-fried 3 fish fingers, grilled 1 pack boil-in-bag cod in butter or parsley sauce 1 Findus Battercrisp Cod Steak, grilled or baked 2 Birds Eye Fish Fingers in Crispy Batter 1 gammon Dalesteak	5 oz (140 g) instant mash 4 oz (115 g) boiled potato 2 croquette potatoes, grilled or baked 3 oz (85 g) boiled noodles 2 oz (55 g) oven chips	Vegetables or salad from unlimited list
2 Findus Crispy Pancakes, any variety except Cheddar 1 Birds Eye Lamb or Beef Grill	4 oz (115 g) boiled potatoes 2 croquette potatoes, grilled or baked 5 oz (140 g) instant mash	

Main meals, quick and easy – 400 calories

Pick one of these	Plus one of these	Plus one of these
1 trimmed chump lamb chop, well grilled	4 oz (115 g) boiled potato	3 tablespoons baked beans
5 oz (140 g) trimmed pork chop, well grilled	4 oz (115 g) potato, mashed with skimmed milk and low-fat spread	3 tablespoons peas
5 oz (140 g) rump or filled steak, well grilled	5 oz (140 g) instant mash	3 tablespoons sweetcorn
1 Quarterpounder, well grilled	2 croquette potatoes baked or grilled	4 oz (115 g) green beans
1 × 6 oz (170 g) breaded haddock portion, baked, grilled or dry-fried		4 oz (115 g) broccoli
1 large chicken portion, baked or grilled		2 rings pineapple
5 oz (140 g) gammon steak, well grilled		4 tablespoons broad beans
2 large sausages, well grilled or dry-fried		
5 oz (140 g) fillet of white fish with 1 portion Cheese Sauce (see recipe page 251) or 4 fl oz (120 ml) from packet made as instructed		
1 Sun Valley Crunchy Chicken portion		
1 Bejam Goldenbake Chicken Breast Steak		
4 oz (115 g) lamb's liver, dry-fried		
1 Birds Eye Liver with onion and Gravy	5 oz (140 g) instant mash with ½ oz (7 g) butter	3 tablespoons peas

Pick one of these	Plus one of these	Plus one of these
1 Bejam Steak Grill 4 chipolatas, well grilled 1 Bejam Chinese Ribsteak 1 Buxted Panbake 1 trout 2 size-3 eggs, dry-fried 1 Ross Indian Chicken Stir-Fry	6 oz (170 g) potato, mashed with skimmed milk and low-fat spread 3 oz (85 g) oven chips 2 hash browns 6 oz (170 g) boiled potato	3 tablespoons sweetcorn 4 oz (115 g) green beans 3 tablespoons baked beans
1 Sainsbury's Seafood and Paella Stir-Fry Chicken	1 portion from 50-calorie fruit selection on page 187	
1 Findus individual Crunchy Cottage Pie	5 oz (140 g) green beans 5 oz (140 g) mixed peas and carrots	
3 tacos filled with ½ × 10 oz (300 g) can beef taco filling + 3 tablespoons taco sauce	chopped salad garnish of choice	

Main meals, quick and easy – 500 calories

Pick one of these	Plus one of these	Plus one of these
5 oz (140 g) gammon steak, grilled 2 size-2 eggs, fried 2 large pork sausages, well grilled or fried 1 large pork sausage, well grilled or fried, + 1 size-3 egg, fried 5 oz (140 g) fillet or rump steak	4 oz (115 g) oven chips 6 oz (170 g) baked potao with ¼ oz (7 g) butter 2 potato waffles 4 oz (115 g) boiled potato, sautéed in non-stick pan in 1 dessertspoon oil 5 oz (140 g) instant mash with ¼ oz (7 g) butter	4 tablespoons peas 4 tablespoons baked beans 4 tablespoons sweetcorn 4 tablespoons broad beans 2 rings pineapple

1 large chicken portion, baked or grilled, plain or Tandoori	1 pitta bread	
1 turkey Cheeseburger		
1 Quarterpounder, grilled		
5 oz (140 g) breaded haddock goujons, baked or grilled		
4 fish fingers, grilled		
2-egg omelette cooked in non-stick pan with ¼ oz (7 g) butter and filled with 2 oz (55 g) chopped mushrooms		
1 Birds Eye Minced Beef and Vegetable Pie	5 oz (140 g) instant mash with ¼ oz (7g) butter	Vegetables or salad from the unlimited list
1 Birds Eye Steak and Kidney Pie	6 oz (170 g) boiled potato	
1 Kraft or Ross individual Steak and Kidney Pudding	3 oz (85 g) oven chips	
1 Chicken Cordon Bleu	3 croquette potatoes, baked or grilled	
1 Chicken Kiev		
1 Safeway Turkey Breast Escalope		
1 Birds Eye Captain's Pie		
1 Birds Eye Fisherman's Choice		
1 Cornish pasty	5 oz (140 g) instant mash	
5 oz (140 g) breaded scampi, baked	4 oz (115 g) oven chips	1 teaspoon tartare sauce

Main meals, quick and easy – 600 calories

Pick one of these	Plus one of these	Plus one of these
6 oz (170 g) steak, fillet or rump, grilled 6 oz (170 g) gammon steak, grilled 3 oz (85 g) liver + 2 rashers lean bacon, grilled 2 large pork sausages, well grilled, and 1 egg 6 oz (170 g) breaded haddock fillet, fried	5 oz (140 g) oven chips 6 oz (170 g) boiled potato, sliced and sautéed in 1 tablespoon oil in non-stick pan	4 oz (115 g) peas 4 oz (115 g) mushrooms, dry-fried 4 oz (115 g) baked beans
1 Chicken Cordon Bleu 1 Chicken Kiev	4 oz (115 g) oven chips 4 oz (115 g) boiled potato, sliced and sautéed in 1 dessertspoon oil in non-stick pan	3 tablespoons peas 4 oz (115 g) green beans

Main meals, heat and serve – 300 calories

Pick one of these	Plus
1 Findus Dinner Supreme Beef Oriental 1 Birds Eye MenuMaster Gammon Steak Platter 1 McCain Complete Meal Italian Chicken	Any 1 portion from the 25-calorie fruit selection on page 186

1 Findus Lean Cuisine Kashmiri Chicken Curry
1 Weightwatchers Chicken in Supreme Sauce with Vegetables
1 Weightwatchers Salmon Mornay with Broccoli
1 Weightwatchers Beef Oriental with Special Egg Rice
1 Bejam Chinese Chicken Stir-Fry
1 Bejam Oriental Beef with rice
1 Bejam Cod and Prawn Pasta
1 Birds Eye Chicken and Seafood Paella
1 Findus Lean Cuisine Cheese Cannelloni

1 McCain Complete Meal Farmhouse Beef
1 St Michael Cottage Pie
1 McCain Complete Meal Farmhouse Chicken
1 Findus Lean Cuisine Chicken and Prawn Cantonese with Noodles
1 Findus Lean Cuisine Cod with White Wine
1 Findus Lean Cuisine Lasagne Verdi

Any 1 portion from the 50-calorie fruit selection on page 187

1 Findus Lean Cuisine Spaghetti Bolognese
1 Bejam Plaice Supreme
1 Bejam Spaghetti Bolognese
1 Tesco Spaghetti Bolognese
1 Safeway Trimrite Chicken Chow Mein

1 Findus Lean Cuisine Beef in Satay Sauce with Oriental Noodles
1 Findus Lean Cuisine Beef and Pork Cannelloni
1 Safeway Trimrite Chicken and Mushrooms with Vegetable Rice
1 Safeway Trimrite Cod Florentine with Vegetables
1 St Michael Chicken Chow Mein

Any 1 portion from the 75-calorie fruit selection on page 187

Main meals, heat and serve — 400 calories

Pick one of these
1 St Michael Beef Enchiladas
1 Birds Eye Roast Beef Platter
1 Birds Eye Chilli con Carne with Rice
1 Birds Eye Chicken à la Crème
1 Birds Eye Beef Curry with Rice
1 Birds Eye Spaghetti Bolognese

Plus
Any 1 portion from the 25-calorie fruit selection on page 186

1 Sharwoods Sweet and Sour Pork with Special Rice 1 Bejam Lasagne Verdi 1 Waitrose Lasagne 1 Sainsbury's Cannelloni Verdi	
1 St Michael Sweet and Sour Chicken with Rice 1 Bejam Roast Beef Platter 1 Bejam Chicken Chasseur with Rice 1 McCain Sweet and Sour Chicken 1 McCain Five-Minute Meal, any variety 1 McCain Pasta Classics, Vegetable Lasagne 1 Findus Dinner Supreme Prawn Curry 1 Birds Eye Mariner's Pasta Gratin 1 Birds Eye Prawn Curry with Rice 1 Birds Eye Roast Turkey Platter	Any 1 portion from the 50-calorie fruit selection on page 187
1 McCain Continental Beef Platter 1 St Michael Seafood Lasagne 1 Sainsbury's Chicken and Ratatouille Bake	Any 1 portion from the 75-calorie fruit selection on page 187

1 Findus Dinner Supreme Beef Madras
1 Findus Dinner Supreme Moussaka
1 Findus Dinner Supreme Chicken Korma
1 Bejam Roast Pork Platter
1 Bejam Smoked Haddock Lasagne
1 Sainsbury's Chicken Curry with Rice
1 St Michael Lasagne
1 Birds Eye Chicken Curry with Rice

Main meals, heat and serve – 500 calories

Pick one of these

1 McCain Beefburger and Chips
1 McCain Farmsteak and Chips
1 McCain Baconburger and Chips
1 McCain Cod and Chips
1 Matthews Beef Curry and Rice
1 Bejam Jumbo Burger and Chips
1 Bejam Beef Curry and Rice
1 Bejam Battered Cod Fingers and Chips
1 St Michael Steak and Kidney Pie meal

Plus

Any 1 portion from the 25-calorie fruit selection on page 186

1 Sainsbury's Grillsteak and Chips
1 Sainsbury's Chicken Nuggets and Chips
1 Sainsbury's Scampi and Chips
1 Birds Eye Prizesteak Platter
1 Birds Eye Oven Crispy Fish and Chips
1 Birds Eye Roast Chicken Platter
1 Asda Lancashire Hotpot
1 Safeway Mash and Bangers
1 Tesco Beef Madras with Rice

1 McCain Gammon and Chips
1 McCain Chicken and Chips
1 Bejam Beef Stroganoff and Rice
1 Bejam Sausage and Mash
1 Bejam Chicken Supreme with Rice
1 St Michael Roast Chicken Meal
1 Sainsbury's Chicken Supreme with Rice
1 Birds Eye Chicken Supreme with Rice
1 Safeway Cod Crumble with Broccoli
1 Waitrose or Asda Potato Dauphinoise

Any 1 portion from the 50-calorie fruit selection on page 187

1 Bejam Curry and Rice 1 Sainsbury's Chicken Lasagne 1 Bejam Roast Chicken platter	Any 1 portion from the 75-calorie fruit selection on page 187
1 Sainsbury's Beef Curry and Rice 1 Bejam Chicken and Chips 1 Safeway Chicken Korma Curry	

Main meals, heat and serve – 600 calories

Pick one of these 1 Tesco Chicken Korma with Rice 1 St Michael Beef Stroganoff with Rice 1 Wiltshire Farms Steak and Kidney Pie with Chips and Peas	*Plus* Any 1 portion from the 25-calorie fruit selection on page 186
1 McCain Cheeseburger and Chips 1 Bejam Battered Sausages and Chips 1 Bejam Sweet and Sour Pork + 1 Bejam Special Fried Rice 1 Safeway Beef Madras Curry with Rice 1 Findus Dinner Supreme Tandoori Chicken Masala	Any 1 portion from the 50-calorie fruit selection on page 187

TOP TAKEAWAYS 300 calories

Choose one of these

1 McDonald's Hamburger with Mild Mustard Sauce (optional)
1 McDonald's Cheeseburger
1 Wimpy Hamburger
1 Wimpy Cheeseburger
1 Wimpy Bacon in a Bun
1 Burger King Hamburger
McDonald's 6 Chicken McNuggets with Barbecue Sauce
1 McDonald's Bacon and Egg McMuffin
1 Lamb Skewer
1 portion Tandoori Chicken
1 average sandwich bar Ham or Egg or Tuna or Chicken
Sandwich, including salad but no mayonnaise

TOP TAKEAWAYS 400 calories

Choose one of these

1 McDonald's Quarterpounder
1 McDonald's Fillet-O-Fish
McDonald's 9 Chicken McNuggets
1 Wimpy Kingsize
1 Wimpy Bacon and Egg in a Bun
1 Burger King Cheeseburger Deluxe
1 Burger King Hamburger Deluxe
1 Doner Kebab
1 Spud U Like Spud 'n One (no butter), Chilli con Carne or
Chicken Curry or Savory Mince or Sausage and Beans or
Tuna Salad variety
1 Pizza Hut Spaghetti Bolognese
1 Chicken Chop Suey
1 Chicken Chow Mein

1 Prawn Chop Suey
1 average sandwich bar Cheese or Bacon Sandwich, or Egg, Tuna or Chicken with mayonnaise

TOP TAKEAWAYS 500 calories

Choose one of these

1 McDonald's Quarterpounder with Cheese
1 McDonald's Sausage and Egg McMuffin
1 McDonald's Scrambled Eggs, Sausage Pattie and Hash Brown
1 Wimpy Quarterpounder
1 Wimpy Chicken in a Bun
1 Wimpy Fish and Chips
1 Wimpy Beanburger
1 Wimpy Hamburger and Chips
1 Burger King Hamburger and Regular French Fries
1 Spud U Like Spud Plus (choice of any two fillings from Chilli con Carne, Chicken Curry, Savoury Mince, Sausage and Beans, Tuna Salad)
1 portion Kentucky Fried Chicken, French Fries, Barbecue Beans
1 portion Chinese Barbecued Spare Ribs
1 Pizza Hut Lasagne
1 Pizza Hut Thin and Crispy Pizza with Sauce and Cheese

TOP TAKEAWAYS 600 calories

Choose one of these

1 McDonald's Big Mac
1 McDonald's Hamburger with Regular French Fries
1 McDonald's Cheeseburger with Regular French Fries
1 Wimpy Quarterpounder with Cheese
1 Wimpy Cheeseburger and Chips
1 Burger King Bacon Double Cheeseburger

1 McDonalds 6 Chicken McNuggets, Regular French Fries, Barbecue Sauce

1 Kentucky Fried Chicken Fillet Burger with Chips and Coleslaw or Beans

1 Kentucky Fried Chicken Dinner for One with Chips and Coleslaw or Beans

1 Pizzaland 10-in Traditional Cheese and Tomato Pizza

1 Pizzaland 10-in Traditional Ham and Mushroom Pizza

TOP TAKEAWAYS 700 calories

Choose one of these

1 McDonald's Quarterpounder with regular French Fries

1 McDonald's 9 Chicken McNuggets and Regular French Fries

1 Burger King Whopper

1 portion fish and chip shop Haddock and Chips

1 portion fish and chip shop Plaice and Chips

1 Chinese Prawns and Mushrooms with Special Fried Rice

1 Chinese Chicken and Vegetables with Special Fried Rice

1 Pizza Hut Thin and Crispy Pizza, Spicy Hot One

1 Pizza Hut Thin and Crispy Pizza, Seafood Supreme

1 Pizza Hut Thin and Crispy Pizza, Supreme

1 Pizzaland 10-in Traditional Pizza, Hot 'n Spicy

1 Pizzaland 10-in Traditional Pizza, Chicken and Sweetcorn

1 Pizzaland 10-in Traditional Pizza, Seafood

1 Pizzaland 7-in Deep Pan Pizza, Cheese and Tomato

1 Deep Pan Pizza Co. Regular Pizza, Polynesia

1 Deep Pan Pizza Co. Regular Pizza, Vegetarian

1 Pizza Express Regular Pizza, Marinara

1 Pizza Express Regular Pizza, Mushroom

TOP TAKEAWAYS 800 calories

Choose one of these

1 McDonald's Quarterpounder with Cheese and Regular
   French Fries

1 Wimpy Quarterpounder with Chips

1 Chicken Curry with Pilau Rice

1 portion fish and chip shop Cod and Chips

1 Pizza Hut Deep Pan Pizza, Spicy Hot One

1 Pizza Hut Thin and Crispy Pizza, Super Supreme

1 Pizzaland 7-in Deep Pan Pizza, Hot 'n Spicy

1 Pizza Express Regular Pizza, Veneziana

1 Pizza Express Regular Pizza, Neptune

1 Deep Pan Pizza Co. Regular Pizza, Hot and Spicy

TOP TAKEAWAYS 900 calories

Choose one of these

1 Pizza Hut Deep Pan Pizza, Seafood Supreme

1 Pizzaland 10-in Traditional Pizza, Passionara

1 Pizzaland 7-in Deep Pan Pizza, Passionara

½ an average set Chinese meal for 2

¼ an average set Chinese meal for 4

1 Sweet and Sour Pork in Batter with Sauce and Special
   Fried Rice

1 Beef with Peppers in Oyster Sauce, 1 Pancake Roll, 1
   Special Fried Rice

1 Beef or Lamb Curry with Rice

VEGETABLES, PASTA AND RICE 25 calories

3 oz (85 g) green beans

2 oz (55 g) beetroot (2 small)

4 oz (115 g) broccoli

4 oz (115 g) sprouts

4 oz (115 g) carrots

4 oz (115 g) swede
4 oz (115 g) macedoine (mixed, chopped vegetables)

VEGETABLES, PASTA AND RICE 50 calories

4 tablespoons baked beans
4 oz (115 g) broad beans
4 oz (115 g) leeks
4 oz (115 g) mangetout peas
4 oz (115 g) parsnips
4 oz (115 g) garden peas
3 oz (85 g) new potatoes
4 oz (115 g) spinach
4 tablespoons sweetcorn
$\frac{1}{2}$ × 10 oz (280 g) can ratatouille

VEGETABLES, PASTA AND RICE 75 calories

3 oz (85 g) red kidney beans (ready-to-eat weight)
4 oz (115 g) sliced courgettes, stir-fried
4 oz (115 g) processed peas
1 medium chunk roast potato
2 croquette potatoes

VEGETABLES, PASTA AND RICE 100 calories

4 oz (115g) Baby Bakes (McCain)
1 potato waffle
2 hash browns
4 oz (115 g) boiled potato
5 oz (140 g) instant mash
4 oz (115 g) potato, mash with skimmed milk and $\frac{1}{4}$ oz (7 g)
   low-fat spread
4 oz (115 g) curried beans with sultanas
4 oz (115 g) mushy peas
4 oz (115 g) butterbeans

4 oz (115 g) mushrooms, stir-fried in 1 dessertspoon oil or
 $\frac{1}{3}$ oz (10 g) butter
1 small onion, sliced and stir-fried in 1 dessertspoon oil
4 oz (115 g) sweet potato
3 oz (85 g) boiled pasta, any kind
3 oz (85 g) boiled rice
1 large chunk roast potato

VEGETABLES, PASTA AND RICE 150 calories

6 oz (170 g) baked potato
4 oz (115 g) potato mashed with whole milk and $\frac{1}{4}$ oz (7 g)
 butter
3 oz (85 g) oven chips
3 oz (85 g) Beefeater chips
3 oz (85 g) sauté potato
5 oz (140 g) boiled rice
5 oz pasta, (140 g) boiled

FRUIT AND JUICES 25 calories

Fruit can be fresh, frozen, cooked (if using sugar, this must
be taken from your Treats allowance) or canned and
drained (weights are given for the drained fruit).
2 fresh apricots
4 oz (115 g) blackberries
4 oz (115 g) blackcurrants
1 clementine
$\frac{1}{2}$ large or 1 small grapefruit
4 oz (115 g) grapefruit segments
2 greengages
1 kiwifruit
3 lychees
1 mandarin
1 average (6 oz, 170 g) slice melon

2 plums
4 oz (115 g) raspberries
4 fl oz (200 ml) tomato juice
6 oz (170 g) rhubarb
1 satsuma
4 oz (115 g) strawberries
1 tangerine

FRUIT AND JUICES 50 calories

Fruit can be fresh, frozen, cooked (if using sugar, this must be taken from your Treats allowance) or canned and drained (weights are given for the drained fruit).
1 apple
4 oz (115 g) canned, drained apricots
4 oz (115 g) cherries
5 dates
4 oz (115 g) gooseberries
4 oz (115 g) grapes
4 oz (115 g) guava
1 nectarine
1 orange
1 ortanique
1 peach or 4 oz (115 g) peach slices, drained
1 pear
2 rings pineapple
4 fl oz (200 ml) orange juice
4 fl oz (200 ml) apple juice with added vitamin C
4 fl oz (200 ml) pineapple juice
4 oz (115 g) fruit salad

FRUIT AND JUICES 75 calories

Fruit can be fresh, frozen, cooked (if using sugar, this must be taken from your Treats allowance) or canned and drained (weights are given for the drained fruit).

1 average banana
1 pomegranate
7 fl oz (200 ml) orange juice
7 fl oz (200 ml) apple juice with added vitamin C
7 fl oz (200 ml) pineapple juice

FRUIT AND JUICES 100 calories

1 whole mango
1 McDonald's Regular Orange Juice

MILK AND YOGURT 50 calories

¼ pint (150 ml) skimmed milk
4 fl oz (120 ml) semi-skimmed milk
⅛ pint (75 ml) whole milk
1 × 4½ oz (125 g) tub diet yogurt (e.g. Shape, Diet Ski)

MILK AND YOGURT 75 calories

⅓ pint (200 ml) skimmed milk
4 fl oz (120 ml) whole milk
1 × 4½ (125 g) tub natural low-fat yogurt

MILK AND YOGURT 100 calories

½ pint (300 ml) skimmed milk
⅓ pint (200 ml) semi-skimmed milk
¼ pint (150 ml) whole milk
70 g (4 level tablespoons) Greek-style yogurt

TREATS, SNACKS AND EXTRAS 25 calories

Sweet Treats

1 heaped teaspoon sugar
2 level teaspoons marmalade, jam, lemon curd or honey
2 sugar lumps
1 Morning Coffee biscuit

Savoury Treats/Extras

1 dessertspoon pickle or chutney of choice
1 dessertspoon tartare sauce or low-calorie salad cream
1 tablespoon tomato ketchup
2 level teaspoons low-fat spread
1 level teaspoon butter or margarine
2 tablespoons thick gravy
2 Oxo cubes in $\frac{1}{2}$ pint (300 ml) water
1 rye crispbread with a little low-fat spread

TREATS, SNACKS AND EXTRAS 50 calories

Sweet Treats

1 level tablespoon golden syrup or honey
2 tablespoons ready-to-eat custard
1 sachet slimmer's instant hot chocolate drink
1 shortcake biscuit
1 diet yogurt
1 × 2$\frac{1}{4}$ oz (75 g) Shape Fromage Frais
Any two treats from 25-calorie section

Savoury Treats

1 poppadom, grilled
1 chipolata sausage, well grilled
1 sachet instant slimmers soup
1 can Weightwatchers soup
Any two treats from 25-calorie list

Extras

$\frac{1}{4}$ oz (7 g) butter or margarine
$\frac{1}{2}$ oz (15 g) low-fat spread
1 tablespoon double or whipped cream
2 tablespoons single or soured cream
1 level tablespoon reduced-calorie mayonnaise

Drinks

1 can alcohol-free lager
1 single measure spirit

TREATS, SNACKS AND EXTRAS 75 calories

Sweet Treats

1 chocolate digestive biscuit
1 Chambourcy Petit Fromage Frais with Fruit Purée
Any three sweet treats from 25-calorie list, or one from 25-
and one from 50-calorie list

Savoury Treats

1 slice bread from a thin-cut loaf with a little low-fat spread
1 oz (30 g) piece pork crackling

Extras

1 tablespoon French dressing
Any three extras from 25-calorie list, or one from 25- and
one from 50-calorie list

TREATS, SNACKS AND EXTRAS 100 calories

Sweet Treats – chocolate and sweets

1 United, orange
1 Jacob's Club wafer
1 McDonalds Yo Yo
2 fingers Kit Kat
1 × $\frac{3}{4}$ oz (20 g) bar Cadbury's Dairy Milk
1 Mars Funsize
1 roll fruit gums
1 roll Polo mints

Sweet Treats – biscuits and cakes

3 Rich Tea biscuits
2 custard creams
2 choc chip cookies

1 Harvest Crunch bar
1 Harvest Chewy bar
1 jam tart
1 mini Swiss roll, jam or chocolate
1 French Fancy

Sweet Treats – desserts and ice cream

1 Birds Eye, Findus or Ross mousse
1 Birds ready-to-eat Instant Whip or Angel Delight
1 Chambourcy Pot au Chocolait
1 Chambourcy Flanby Caramel
2 oz (55 g) vanilla, strawberry, choc or raspberry ripple ice
   cream + 1 wafer
1 French-style set yogurt
5½ oz (150 g) pot Ambrosia low-fat rice pudding
5½ oz (150 g) pot Ambrosia low-fat custard
1 soft ice cream cone, standard
¼ pint (150 ml) jelly + 1 dessertspoon single cream

Drinks

½ pint (300 ml) beer, lager (light) or cider
1 × 5 fl oz (150 ml) glass dry or medium wine
1 double measure spirit (any) with calorie-free mixer
   (optional)
11½ fl oz (330 ml) can lemonade, orangeade or cherryade
½ pint (300 ml) orange or lemon squash or blackcurrant
   cordial

Savouries

1 pack Lower Fat Crisps, cheese and onion flavour
1 pack Ringos
1 pack Quavers
1 can Weightwatchers soup with 2 crispbreads

Extras

1 slice bread from a medium-cut loaf with low-fat spread

1 slice bread from a thin-cut loaf with butter
½ oz (15 g) butter
1 oz (30 g) low-fat spread
5 tablespoons boiled rice
2 oz (55 g) oven chips
4 oz (115 g) boiled or baked potato
1 level tablespoon mayonnaise
1 size-3 egg, dry-fried
1 large chunk roast potato
2 oz (55 g) lean meat
1½ oz (45 g) Yorkshire pudding
1 oz (30 g) pastry

TREATS, SNACKS AND EXTRAS 150 calories

Sweet Treats – chocolate and sweets

1 oz (30 g) banana chips
1 stick pack Fox's Glacier Fruits or Mints
1 single Milky Way
1 single Twix Teabreak bar

Sweet Treats – biscuits and cakes

1 Wagon Wheel
1 Bird's Eye Dairy Cream Eclair
1 chocolate cup cake
1 cherry slice

Sweet Treats – desserts and ice cream

1 Bird's Eye Supermousse
1 Chambourcy Black Forest Dessert
1 Eden Vale Black Forest Trifle
1 Eden Vale Raspberry or Strawberry Trifle
1 St Ivel Fruit Trifle
1 Lyons Maid Cornish Vanilla Cup
1 Lyons Maid Dark Satin Choc Ice

1 Walls Choc Bar, dark and golden or golden vanilla

Savouries
1 oz (30 g) Cheddar and 1 crispbread
1 standard bag crisps

Drinks
⅓ pint (200 ml) hot chocolate drink made with semi-skimmed milk and 2 teaspoons cocoa or drinking chocolate
1 × ⅓ pint (200 ml) carton milk shake
1 can Coca-Cola
1 sachet instant Horlicks or hot chocolate
½ pint (300 ml) strong lager or beer

TREATS, SNACKS AND EXTRAS 200 calories

Sweet Treats – chocolate and sweets
1 Bar Six
1 × 1½ oz (40 g) bar Cadbury's Dairy Milk
1 Cadbury's Creme Egg
1 Wispa
1 Fry's Chocolate Cream
1 × 1½ oz (38 g) bag Maltesers
1 roll pack Toffos
1 Crunchie
1 Choc Chip Tracker (1½ oz, 40 g)

Sweet Treats – biscuits and cakes
1 snack-pack shortcake biscuits
1 United Extra Time
1 mince pie
1 mini apple pie
1 blackcurrant sundae
1 cherry bakewell tart
1 jam doughnut
1 teacake

1 scone
1 croissant

Sweet Treats – desserts and icecream
1 individual cheesecake
1 St Ivel Black Forest Gateau
1 Eden Vale Chocolate Supreme
1 Birds Eye Arctic Circle
1 King Cone, chocolate, strawberry or vanilla
1 Cornetto, strawberry or choc 'n nut
1 Thick and Creamy yogurt
1 Greek yoghurt (4½ oz, 125 g)

Savouries
1 × 1½ oz (40 g) pack mixed nuts and raisins
1 × 1½ oz (40 g) pack peanuts, any kind
1 average corn on the cob with ½ oz (15 g) butter

TREATS, SNACKS AND EXTRAS 300 calories
Sweet treats
1 average portion apple pie and custard
1 average portion Black Forest Gateau with cream
1 Bounty twin
1 Twix twin
1 Milky Way twin
1 Standard Mars bar
1 biscuit and raisin Yorkie
1 Cadbury's fruit and nut standard bar

Savoury treats
1 bag popcorn
1 bag tortilla chips
1 × 2 oz (55 g) bag roasted peanuts

9 · EATING OUT – AND DAYS OFF

It is a rare diet book that treats slimmers like ordinary human beings who actually want to do normal things occasionally, like go out for a meal, visit friends for supper or even take a holiday.

However, I know that you *do* have a life B.D. (beyond diet), and if I don't recognize that fact, your slimming success will suffer.

£8·2 billion and rising is spent every year on eating out in Britain, excluding takeaways. That's over £3 a head for every man, woman and child every week. In reality, though, we're divided into two groups – people who eat out very frequently, usually because of their work, and people who eat out only occasionally, usually for social reasons. Depending upon which group you come into, we have to apply different tactics.

· FREQUENT FEASTING ·

Let's be realistic. If you are in the habit of eating out every day (or nearly every day), be it a trucker's roadside café or a five-star restaurant, there's no point me kidding you that you can eat as much as you like and still lose weight. These meals were probably the very reason you put on weight in the first place, and trying to diet around them without making any changes is going to be almost impossible. The reasons for this are:

• Chefs, whether they are the egg and chips brigade or the haute-cuisine school, rarely give a thought to how many calories their concoctions contain. Canteen and café-style meals are often high in surplus fat that you would have avoided had you been cooking the same meals yourself the Junk Food Diet way. International and upmarket eating places tend to provide everything coated with rich sauces or swamped in butter.

• Portion sizes are often large, especially in cafés and canteens. So, even if what you have on your plate isn't a particularly high-calorie food, the amount you're given turns it into a high-calorie plateful.

• Restaurants need to make a profit – and they stand more chance of doing that if you eat three courses rather than one. Add to that the temptation of 'free' fodder such as roll and butter, or after-meal sweets, or crisps, and it's so easy to eat far more than you ever intended.

• Your own natural greed. If you are eating at home and three-quarters of the way through the meal you have had enough, you will probably leave the rest. In a café or restaurant, you are much more likely to think, 'If I've paid for it, I'm damn well going to eat it.' And how about if someone *else* is paying? Then the temptation to eat all you can cram in is even stronger.

• If you eat out, you drink.

So my first thought for you to ponder on is, are all these meals out really necessary? Could you not take a packed lunch to work instead, or on the road if you have to travel? Could you not get by with a takeaway sandwich at this time of day, and have your main meal when you do get home?

If you come to the conclusion that there genuinely is no way round your eating-out dilemma, then what we have to do is attempt to bring the calorie content of all those meals down to an acceptable level within your diet.

First, then, here are some general guidelines for you to follow:

- Follow the Pick Your Own Plan rather than the Set Diet, and treat your meal out as your main meal of the day.
- If you have a choice of where to eat, go for somewhere that has several items on its menu that are plain, straightforward dishes in which it is hard to 'hide' calories. On a daily basis, for instance, Chinese, Indian and cordon bleu restaurants are lethal.
- Always keep the Junk Food Diet rules in your mind when you're eating out. For instance, cut visible fat off meat and stop eating when you're full.
- If possible, pick an eaterie that is happy for you to have your vegetables without butter garnish; your 'grilled' fish really grilled and not coated in butter.
- Eat your fill of plain cooked vegetables or salad, and again, ask for them all ungarnished or without dressing. Remember, not all vegetables are low in calories – fried onion rings or mushrooms and all kinds of fried potatoes are high in calories.
- Try some forward planning. Decide what you're going to eat beforehand if possible so you needn't be tempted by the menu.
- Use your common sense. Despite all my warnings, you *can* eat a reasonable dieter's meal in any restaurant if you're sensible. Just remember that the most fattening foods are fats, and things containing fat, such as pastry, oily sauces like mayonnaise and Hollandaise, vinaigrette, and deep-fried small items like whitebait. However, a little of one or two high-cal items is probably all right. Use your common sense!

Right, armed with these guidelines, here's what you do next. You'll remember that your main meal should be no more than 500 calories if you're on 1,000 calories a day, or 600 calories if you're dieting on 1,250 or 1,500 calories a day. With the help of the meal listings at the end of this chapter, you simply pick your meal to the correct total, or less. Then make sure that the rest of what you eat on the same day doesn't add up to more than your allowed calorie total.

If you want to use your daily Treats calories on an extra with your meal, such as a drink, a dessert or some butter, then do so – but remember, you'll be leaving yourself with not many calories left for the rest of the day.

You will find it hard to pick a three-course meal in a restaurant and still stay within your 5- or 600-calorie limit. I don't believe you really *need* three courses anyway, but you could, if you are determined, have a dessert as your daily treat.

The only way you can be really sure that you're doing okay is to ask yourself the pertinent question . . . am I still losing weight?

· INFREQUENT FEASTING ·

Celebrations are what make life worthwhile. Whether it's a birthday, a wedding, a new job or a holiday – everyone needs something to celebrate now and then. But celebration means food and drink.

At such times, there is only one thing worse than having to say, 'Sorry, I can't eat that/drink that/come out with you – I'm on a diet', and that is hearing someone else say it instead. When people want to have a good time, diet bores are deadly.

So the next time that happens to you, don't even think about sticking to your diet. I give you leave to eat what you want without feeling guilty. And that's important. If you feel guilty, not only will you not enjoy yourself but you'll also feel so bad afterwards that you'll abandon your diet.

The reason there is no need to feel guilty is that I have a very simple way for you to indulge without ruining your slimming campaign. It's a system called the Treats Transfer.

The Treats Transfer

Why is it that when you sit down for a slap-up meal with a friend, you eat less than she does, and yet she is slim and you are not?

It is probably quite simply that she, without even thinking about it, obeys the first law of eating: balance. She'll eat trillions of calories tonight, but tomorrow she may eat very little. In other words, she quite naturally practises the calorie common sense that overweight people tend to ignore.

You must learn *not* to ignore it – and by practising the Treats Transfer, you can. Here's how it works.

Fact one: whichever calorie level you're dieting on, you have a daily treats allowance of either 100, 200 or 300 calories a day. Fact two: if you're going out somewhere special for a meal or party or day out, you almost always know well in advance.

All you have to do is cut down a little on your food intake for a while before your special event by 'saving' those treats calories rather than 'spending' (eating) them.

Now, although you may not know exactly what you're going to eat on your celebration, I can tell you that at any one meal, if you are an 'average' person, you will eat no more than 1,500 calories at most. You may get through far less, even including alcohol. On the other hand, you may know exactly what you will eat – for instance, that you will have, if it's available, prawn cocktail, plus bread, chicken Kiev and Black Forest gateau, together with a few glasses of wine. Now, I can tell you from looking up the lists I compiled at the end of this chapter, that that little lot will come to around 1,400 calories.

Now, say you're on the 1,250 calories a day diet. On the day you are due to go out for this meal, you have a 200-calorie breakfast and a 300-calorie lunch plus 100 calories for fruit and milk. That leaves you with 650 calories left towards your evening out, which means you have to find an extra 750 calories from somewhere. Easy! All you do is forgo your daily treat of 200 calories a day for four days beforehand. Then you can go out, eat your favourite meal, drink your wine, and not need to feel one tiny bit guilty, because you know you aren't doing any damage to your diet. Good, isn't it?

You try some more possible combinations yourself. Make up some meals you'd really like, work out how many surplus calories you need to borrow, and see how few days it takes for you to 'earn' them. It's a very reassuring pastime.

You can use the Treats Transfer in other ways: for a cream tea out shopping with friends, or a whole day off your diet every Sunday, say. All you ever have to do is work out roughly what your night or day 'off' is going to 'cost', and allow for it. It's always best to 'save up' in advance, rather than trying to pay back your calorie bank after the event. Paying for something after you've had it is always harder; the incentive of something to look forward to has gone.

I would also suggest that you practise the Treats Transfer as an occasional thing – no more than once a week, otherwise you'll get in a muddle with your figures. And once you get in a muddle, you are likely to start cheating.

How do you know you're doing okay? If you're losing weight, you're doing all right.

· CHRISTMAS AND HOLIDAYS ·

Lastly, a word or two about celebrations that go on longer than an evening or a day ... your annual holiday, say, or Christmas.

My advice is for you to treat yourself like a normal person, and behave like one, which means eating what you fancy in moderation most of the time, having the odd blow-out, and *also having times when you can leave food alone because there's something better going on.*

Think of food as part of your break/holiday, not the be-all and end-all of it.

If you try the alternative, carrying on with your diet while all around you eat, drink and are merry, you're handing yourself a recipe for disaster – a battle on your plate.

With a relaxed attitude, okay, you may put on a couple of pounds during the break; you certainly won't lose much. But afterwards you can get back to steady weight loss with no real damage done.

· EATING-OUT GUIDE ·

(All calorie counts are approximate unless stated otherwise)

Café/Canteen meals

Breaded fish and chips	700
Double egg and chips	650
1 sausage, 1 egg and chips	650
2 sausages, beans and chips	750
2 sausages, beans and mash	500
Plain omelette with salad	300
Plain omelette and chips	650
Ham salad	300
Quiche salad	500
Egg mayonnaise salad	400
Steak pie, mash and vegetables	700
1 portion salad cream	50
1 portion mayonnaise	100
Lasagne	600
Moussaka (10 oz, 285 g)	550
Cottage pie (10 oz, 285 g)	350

Little Chef (roadside cafés)

(Calorie counts are exact)

Early Starter	765
American-style Breakfast	650
Plaice and Chips	745
Cod and Chips	700
Quarterpound Burger	468
Quarterpound Burger with Chips	875
Gammon Steak Platter	800
Chicken Platter	590
Vegetable side order (no butter)	119
Side Salad + Potato	250
Big Choice Chicken	879
Prawn Salad	446

Steak Sandwich	258
Chicken as a Snack	260
2 Sugar and Lemon Pancakes	245

Bar Meals

Average Ploughman's Lunch	550
Average cheese sandwich	350
Average ham roll	300
Scampi in a basket (no chips)	500
Beef curry with boiled rice	500
Baked potato with butter and grated cheese	450

Restaurants
English/International

Consommé	30
Grapefruit cocktail	50
Fruit juice	50
Melon	40
Vegetable soup	100
Cream soup, any kind	150
Prawn cocktail	210
Thin slice bread and butter	100
Liver pâté with toast and butter	300
Smoked mackerel pâté with toast and butter	300
Avocado vinaigrette	385
Avocado with prawns in mayonnaise	450
Deep-fried mushrooms	300
Roll, plain	120
Roll with butter	200

Roast meat platter including potatoes, etc.	500–600
Fillet steak, 6 oz (170 g), well done	220
Rump steak, 8 oz (225 g), well done	340
Sole, grilled, without butter	450
Plaice (unbreaded), grilled, without butter	250
Half a chicken, including skin	450
Chicken Kiev with vegetables	600
3 lean lamb cutlets	300
Trout with almonds	500
Gammon steak, 6 oz (170 g), grilled	300
Breaded seafood platter	450
¼ roast duck with sauce	500
Scampi provençale and rice	400–500
Average (5 oz, 140 g) portion chips	350
Average portion boiled potatoes	125
Average portion fried mushrooms	120
Average portion onion rings	150
Average jacket potato with butter	300
Average jacket potato without butter	200
Ice cream	120
Fresh fruit, per piece	50
Fresh fruit salad	100
Sorbet	90
Creme caramel	150
Strawberries or raspberries, sugar and cream	200
Average serving cream	100
Black Forest gateau	300
Apple pie	300
Trifle	300
Average serving cheese and biscuits, butter	300–400

Berni Inns

(Calorie counts are exact)

5 oz (140 g) rump steak, well done	215
6 oz (170 g) fillet steak, well done	220
8 oz (225 g) sirloin steak, well done	330
12 oz (340 g) sirloin steak, well done	490
14 oz (400 g) T-bone steak, well done	445
Gammon steak with pineapple	329
6 oz (170 g) scampi	480
1 serving barbecue sauce	70
1 serving Diane sauce	50
1 serving au poivre sauce	60
1 serving chasseur sauce	30
1 serving Bearnaise sauce	360
Butter portion	70
Jacket potato	180
5 oz (140 g) French fries	230
3 oz (85 g) peas	50
3 oz (85 g) green beans	20
Onion rings	160
Mushrooms	120
Ice cream	120
Apple pie and cream	418
Fantasy Island	310
Sherry trifle	400

Italian

Minestrone soup	200
Mozzarella cheese and tomato salad	200
Risotto	600
Spaghetti Bolognese	600
Spaghetti Napoletana	450

Cannelloni	700
Garlic-butter-stuffed chicken with vegetables	800
Tagliatelle with cream and ham	400
Veal escallope with vegetables	600

Greek

Taramasalata, 2 oz (55 g) serving	270
Hummus, 2 oz (55 g) serving	100–150
1 pitta bread	180
Stuffed Vine Leaves as starter (3 leaves)	150–200
Stuffed Vine Leaves with Rice (main course)	600
1 Lamb Kebab stick with Vegetables and Rice	450
1 average portion Kleftico (baked lamb) and Salad	400
1 Greek Salad with Fetta, including olive oil	250
Moussaka, 14 oz (400 g)	770

Chinese

Barbecued spare ribs	400–500
Shark's Fin Soup	90
Chicken Chop Suey	400
Chicken Chow Mein	400
¼ of an average set Chinese meal for 4	900

Mexican restaurant

3 Tacos with Beef Filling and Sauce	350
Enchiladas, average serving	600
Chilli con Carne with Rice	600
Chilli con Carne with Baked Potato	550
Chilli starter with Tortilla Chips	350

Guacamole, average serving	130
Tostada with Refried Beans	150

Indian

Chicken Tikka starter	300
Chicken Tandoori, 1 piece	250
Onion Bhaji starter	200
Samosa starter	200
Average Chicken Curry, no rice	500
Average Chicken Tikka or Tandoori Masala, no rice	500
Average Chicken Korma, no rice	700
Average Beef Curry, no rice	600
Average Lamb Curry, no rice	600
Average Vegetable Curry, no rice	400
Prawn Biriani	600
Average Madras Curry, no rice	500
Average portion Pilau Rice	300
Average portion Boiled Rice	150
1 poppadom	60
1 naan	300
1 chapati	150
1 cucumber raita, average serving	30
1 dessertspoon mango chutney	25

Fast Food Restaurants
McDonald's

(*Calorie counts are exact*)	
Hamburger (regular)	252
Cheeseburger	300
Quarterpounder	**404**

Quarterpounder with Cheese	496
Big Mac	552
Filet-O-Fish	416
6 Chicken McNuggets	270
9 Chicken McNuggets	407
Barbeque Sauce	46
Sweet Curry Sauce	55
Mild Mustard Sauce	54
Sweet and Sour Sauce	44
Regular French Fries	288
Large French Fries	385
Apple Pie	250
Regular cola	96
Diet Cola	0
Regular Orange Drink	115
Regular Root Beer	127
Vanilla Milkshake	357
Milk	166
Big Breakfast	642
Bacon and Egg McMuffin	311
Sausage and Egg McMuffin	511

Wimpy

(Calorie counts are exact)

Hamburger	260
Cheeseburger	305
Quarterpounder	540
Quarterpounder with cheese	585
Kingsize	410
Chicken in a Bun	485
Fish and Chips	460
Beanburger	520
Bacon in a Bun	280

Bacon and Egg in a Bun	425
Chips	265
Milkshake	255
Apple Pie	315

Burger King

(Calorie counts are exact)

Bacon Double Cheeseburger	600
Cheeseburger	360
Cheeseburger Deluxe	410
Chicken in a Bun	690
Crispy Cod in a Bun	540
Double Burger	430
Hamburger	310
Whopper	670
Whopper with Cheese	760
French Fries, Regular	210
French Fries, Large	330
Apple Pie	330
Milkshake	340

Pizzaland

(Calorie counts are exact)
10-in Traditional Pizzas (serve 1)

Cheese and Tomato	608
Chicken and Sweetcorn	693
Seafood	695
Ham and Pineapple	709
Passionara	885
Hot 'n Spicy	708
Vegetarian	841

Ham and Mushroom	619

7-in Deep Pan Pizzas (serve 1), or $\frac{1}{2}$ × 10-in Deep Pan

Cheese and Tomato	649
Chicken and Sweetcorn	747
Seafood	742
Ham and Pineapple	742
Passionara	894
Hot 'n Spicy	793
Vegetarian	700
Ham and Mushroom	729

Pizza Hut

(Calorie counts are exact)

Pizzas, small (serve 1)	Thin and Crispy	Pan
Sauce and Cheese	458	715
Vegetarian	620	734
Spicy Hot One	722	780
Seafood Supreme	683	877
Supreme	643	830
Super Supreme	761	966
Priazzos, small (serve 1–2)		
Roma		989
Florentine		1,042
Verona		1,002
Main-course Pastas		
Lasagne		529
Spaghetti Bolognese		395
Tagliatelle Verdi Vegetarian		600
Tagliatelle Supreme		684
Salads		
Mixed regular, no dressing		140
Mixed regular, with dressing		338

Deep Pan Pizza Co.

(Calorie counts are exact)

Standard Burger with Coleslaw and Baked Potato	870
Standard Burger with Coleslaw and Fries	975
Slenderizer Burger	395
Quarter Chicken with Coleslaw and Baked Potato	830
Pizzas, regular (serve 1)	
Polynesian	710
Vegetarian	660
Hot and Spicy	820
Meat Treat	880

Garfunkels

Average main course help-yourself salad	450
Spaghetti with tomato sauce	350
Omelette with baked potato	450
Quiche with salad bar	500
Burger with mixed salad, no bun, baked potato	500
Grilled sirloin with baked potato	500
¼ roast chicken and help yourself from salad bar	450
Chicken kebab with salad bar	400
Chicken kebab with barbecue sauce and rice	400
Salad bar – average values	
Green salad, average serving	10
Tomato salad, average serving	10
Peppers, 1 spoonful	5
Beetroot, 1 spoonful	15
Sweetcorn salad, 1 spoonful	25
Potato salad, 1 spoonful	40
Pasta salad, 1 spoonful	40
Coleslaw, 1 spoonful	30

Carrots and nut salad, 1 spoonful	25
Bean salad, 1 spoonful	35
Mushrooms à la Grecque, 1 spoonful	50
Deep-fried aubergine slice, 1	75
Deep-fried mushroom, 1	50
Hard-boiled egg, 1 half	40
Pilchard in tomato sauce, 1	50
Grated cheese, 1 spoonful	60
Cottage cheese, 1 spoonful	25
Rice salad, 1 spoonful	40
Cold chicken wing, 1	40
Tuna mayonnaise, 1 spoonful	50

Tea shop

1 average slice gateau	300
1 average slice rich chocolate cake	350
1 scone with jam and cream	300
1 toasted teacake with butter	200
1 fancy sponge cake	200
Egg on toast	230
Beans on toast	220

· A SUMMARY OF WHAT YOU'VE READ IN CHAPTER 9 ·

· If you eat out regularly, you need to recognize that these meals should be controlled.
· You can get a reasonably low-calorie meal almost anywhere if you really want to.
· If you eat out infrequently, go ahead and enjoy yourself.
· Don't bother dieting on holiday.

10 · SUCCESS!
NOW KEEP SLIM FOR LIFE

Well done! You lost those surplus pounds – or stones – with your own determination (and a little help from me), so you have every right to feel pleased with yourself. It wasn't *that* hard, was it?

Now comes the even more important bit. Staying slim.

It is a fact that most people find keeping the weight off harder than losing it. It is a fact that two-thirds of dieters put some or all of their weight back on sooner or later. For most, it's within a year of getting slim.

What a terrible waste of effort! I want to make sure you are not one of those people.

· PRACTICALITIES ·

To begin with, let's deal with the immediate, pleasant task of getting you off your low-calorie diet and back on to a non-slimming, but non-fattening, one.

Thanks to the Junk Food Diet, two of the most common problems dieters face when they come back to a normal diet won't apply to you.

First, be glad you didn't follow a fad diet – a liquids-only diet, say, or a grapefruit and fish diet, for example. Those are the diets that do nothing whatsoever for you long-term, because they don't teach you long-term sensible eating habits that you can live with. Having slimmed on the Junk Food Diet, you will easily make the transition back to a

213

normal diet because 'normal' will be almost identical to the slimming diet – only there will be more of it . . .

Second, be glad you didn't crash diet – lose weight too quickly. It's a fact that weight lost quickly comes back quickly. On the Junk Food Diet, you had plenty to eat and you lost weight gradually.

So, with those two plusses, you have a head start in the staying-slim game. Now, how best to cash in? First, I'll explain a couple of things you should know about what happens when you start eating *more* after a period of eating *less*.

Remember when you began dieting how I explained to you that three pounds or so of the initial, high, first week's weight loss would be fluid, not fat? Well, when you step up your food intake the fluid levels in your body also adjust, but this time you gain fluid (and carbohydrate) rather than lose it. You may, indeed, gain those three pounds back again. This is *not* fat, it is fluid. It is the same fluid that causes people to say, guiltily and almost unbelievingly, after they've eaten just one big meal, 'I've put on pounds!' The more you eat, the more fluid your body retains. It's normal, healthy functioning. In other words, if you finish dieting at, say, 9 stone, the fluid increase will mean you level out at between 9 stone 2 lb and 9 stone 4 lb. However, because of the way in which we're going to get you up to your maintenance diet level, this fluid gain won't be an overnight thing; it will be gradual. And, because we will be building up your calorie level gradually too, you will find that you probably lose another pound or two of fat before we get you up to maintenance over the next six weeks or so – so that the extra fat loss will balance out the fluid gain – and you'll still end up 9 stone (or whatever).

The next thing you should know is that people who tell

you they have to stay on a strict low-calorie diet for life in order to stay slim are exaggerating grossly.

Unless you're foolishly trying to maintain a weight that's far too low for your height, that just isn't true. On the other hand, it is true to say that you can't go back to eating as much as you did when you were overweight. This is for two reasons. One, eating that much made you fat. Eating that much again will make you fat again. Two, remember I explained to you that a 16-stone man needs more to eat than a 9-stone woman to maintain his weight. And you, at, say, 9 stone, need less food to maintain your new size than you did at, say, 11 stone.

So, please, don't feel cheated or hard done by that you can't go back to eating however much it was that you were eating.

What you *will* be able to do is eat a reasonably normal amount for a person of normal weight. According to Ministry of Agriculture statistics, women aged between eighteen and fifty-four carrying out most occupations need around 2,150 calories a day to maintain normal bodyweight, but the figure for different age groups and levels of activity varies from 1,680 up to 2,500. Men in most occupations between ages eighteen and thirty-four need around 2,900 and men between thirty-five and sixty-four need 2,750 – but again, the figures for men of different age groups and occupations varies from 2,150 up to 3,350.

What all this means is that although it is likely that you will need somewhere around 2,150 if you are female or 2,750–2,900 if you're male, these figures are only a guide. Everyone is different, and just as you slimmed on the level that was right for *you*, so your maintenance level will be specific to you and may be different from your friend's.

So please don't feel too bad if you happen to be the

woman or man who needs fewer calories than your next-door neighbour. What other people eat is no concern of yours. You must eat what you need for your own body.

If you are one of the minority of people who don't need many calories a day – say, you find your maintenance level is only 1,700 – you can, if you wish, speed your metabolic rate (your calorie-consuming system) up with a few crafty tactics. You can step up the amount of aerobic exercise you do – walking, cycling and so on. You can build up the amount of muscle in your body (by a daily workout with light weights, for instance), because muscle burns up calories more quickly than other body tissue. And you can eat several snack meals a day rather than one or two bigger meals, because this speeds up your metabolic rate a little too.

But, looking on the positive side, even if you do need slightly fewer calories than your friend, the fact is that you can still eat more than when you were dieting without getting fat again. Considerably more. Anybody who says otherwise is not telling the truth. What we have to do is discover what that amount is.

· THE TRANSITION PERIOD ·

Because neither you nor I can predict your calorie maintenance requirements exactly, the only safe way to start eating more is to build up your food intake gradually. Here, step by step, is what you do.

Week One

Whatever you do, do not get on the scales, say, 'Yippee! I did it!', and go on a week-long binge. If you do, you'll have wasted the very considerable asset your diet has given you: the fact that less is now normal. You are used to smaller amounts; don't give your stomach or your brain the chance to get back into the habit of eating a lot more straight away.

Instead, do this. Whatever dieting calorie level you finished on, add on 250 calories, so that each day this week you eat 1,250 if you were on 1,000, 1,500 if you were on 1,250 and 1,750, if by any chance, you finished your diet still on 1,500 calories. (If you did, you're probably male.) Carry on as before, picking your food from the listings in Chapter 8. Make sure the extra calories aren't sweet treats, though. Stick to your new calorie level throughout Week One. You may notice a small *fluid* weight gain.

Weeks Two and Three

Add a further 250 calories to your diet. For these two weeks, your level will now be either 1,500, 1,750 or 2,000, again made up from the meal choices in the Pick Your Own listings, but not from the sweet treats (once you've used up the maximum treats allowance of 300 calories).

Nobody I know of will yet have reached the stage where they are gaining weight. (If you are on 2,000 calories a day now, it is because you were still slimming on 1,500). A further weight gain due to fluid may occur.

Weeks Four and Five

Add on another 250 calories. So for these two weeks, you will be on either 1,750, 2,000 or 2,250. A few of you may have reached your maintenance level by now, but this won't become obvious until Week Six. Fluid weight gain should have ceased.

Week Six onwards

Now start adding in blocks of 100 calories more each week. So for Week Six, you are on either 1,850, 2,100 or 2,350 calories a day, Week Seven you are on 1,950, 2,200 or 2,450, and so on. At this stage you should weigh yourself once a week at the same time with no clothes on, on the same scales. If there's no weight gain (assuming, for women, you aren't pre-period), add another 100 calories for another week then weigh yourself again.

Sooner or later (it will probably be sooner now), you will get on the scales and find you've put on $\frac{1}{2}$ a pound or a pound. This will not be fluid; it will be fat. That means that you've passed your maintenance level, and it's time to go back to the level you were on last week. Say, you've spent a week on 2,200 and you've gained. Go back to 2,100. That is your permanent maintenance level.

That is not to say that you should eat exactly 2,100 calories (for example) every day for the rest of your life. Some days you will eat a bit more, some a bit less; some weeks you'll eat more, some less. But, if you average out at that amount over a period of time, you will never put on weight again – except by getting much older (we need about 50 calories a day less for every five years older we get over the age of thirty).

Don't skip on doing this climb up to your maintenance level. I repeat, levels vary so much from person to person that I can't tell you what yours will be. What you want is control of the situation – and this way, you have it.

· YOUR MAINTENANCE DIET ·

Having found your correct calorie level, you can stick to it simply by following the Junk Food Diet principles. Just pick a wide variety of meals and foods from the listings in Chapter 8 up to your new calorie level. You can supplement this diet with foods from the Junk Food Directory (see page 282) and by buying other foods with their calorie content on the pack, and you can buy a comprehensive calorie counter, like the *Slimmer's Complete Guide to Calories*, for around £1 and include many, many more foods in your diet.

Remember the tips that helped you to slim are the ones that will help you stay slim; don't waste calories on high-calorie foods when low-calorie ones would do just as well; and don't forget those crafty ways to cut the fat out of your diet.

I'm not saying you should spend the rest of your life counting calories. Far from it. But if you keep an eye on what you eat, bearing in mind your known calorie maintenance level, you won't get fat again.

Here are some more tips to help you stay slim and healthy:

- Eat a varied diet.
- Don't eat mindlessly: be aware of what you're eating and always ask yourself, 'Do I really need this?'
- Let hunger be your main reason for eating.
- Several small snacks a day rather than a few big meals will keep you from ever getting too hungry and will help your metabolic rate.
- Put small to medium portions on your plate rather than big ones. For instance, if you're serving potatoes and are not sure whether to give yourself two pieces or three, have two. If you're still genuinely hungry at the end of your meal, you can always have some more.
- Smaller plate and dish sizes will help you control your portion sizes.

· Build your favourite foods into your diet so that you never feel deprived.

· Eat slowly. If you eat too fast, you'll tend to finish your meal still feeling falsely hungry. That's where foods that need some chewing, like fibre-rich vegetables, help.

· Never let yourself get so hungry that you'll eat anything and everything in sight.

· Continue with the Junk Food Diet policy on sweet treats: have no more than 300 calories' worth a day, or 2,100 a week.

· Weigh yourself once a week, no more, no less, at the same time of day with no clothes on, on the same scales.

So there you have all the practical advice you really need to stay slim for ever. But you're only human, and I would like to forearm you with some sensible advice on what to do should the unthinkable happen and you find you have put on a little weight.

· THE THIN END OF THE WEDGE ·

For most of us, weight slips back on gradually. We lead busy lives, perhaps we stop being quite so careful during a particularly busy time, perhaps we don't weigh ourselves for a while – and then we discover the truth. In fact, we might have put on so much weight that it's diet time again, and what a daunting prospect it can be second time around.

This is exactly what I want you to avoid. So I want you to promise me that, without getting obsessive about it, you *will* weigh yourself once a week, after what you consider a normal day's eating – not after a celebration blow-out, for instance. (And, for women, not just before a period.)

If you get on the scales at this weekly weigh-in and find you have put on a couple of pounds, don't panic. And don't get dispirited. That sounds like a fat person's thinking. And you're not a fat person.

No, what you do is remember that you're a *normal* person. And what do normal people do when they have put on a couple of pounds? They cut back a little for a day or two, and lose it. So that's what you do.

If you need the security of a regulated plan, then go back on the Junk Food Diet, 1,500 calories level, either the Set Diet or the Pick Your Own Plan, for around a week.

If you don't need that much structure, simply put small portions of the higher-calorie foods on your plate and make up the spaces with bigger portions of the low-calorie ones.

What you don't want to do is ignore that couple of pounds, hoping they'll go away of their own accord. Again, that's a fat person thinking. And they won't. Unless you do something about them straight away, what they *will* do is cunningly turn into half a stone. If you then decide you can live with that for a while, that pound or two will be nearer a stone, and at some stage you will have to make the decision: do I diet again or go on getting fatter?

You should *never* put on more than three or four pounds without doing something about it straight away.

If I have to pick the single most important factor that will help you to stay slim for life without hassle, it's this: *don't* let yourself get more than a few pounds over the weight you feel best at, ever. Anything more is the thin end of the wedge.

· BEING A SLIM PERSON ·

I leave you with some last words of advice which I hope you won't need. There are some people, probably a lot more than you'd imagine, who never really feel like slim people even if they succeed in dieting. This doesn't just happen to very obese people or to people who have been seriously overweight for years. It can also happen to people who always want to be a stone or so less than they are.

It's a great temptation, if you've been plagued in one way or another by your weight for years, to feel that even though you've slimmed this time, your size is beyond your control. You *know* what to do to stay slim, but you don't *do* it. Somewhere deep down you feel that your larger size is the real you, your slim self an impostor.

So listen – you aren't a fat person wearing a temporary slim body. You are a slim person. When you were fat you were a slim person in a fat person's body. And don't let anyone tell you otherwise. (I've known successful slimmers who really did put weight back on again because jealous friends or selfish relatives persuaded them to.)

So please remember that you and only you are responsible for your own size. You weren't meant to be fat; no one is *meant* to be fat. You can't alter your natural height, your frame size or even a natural tendency to put on weight while eating the same as your slim cousin – but you don't have to be fat; you *can* keep the weight off. You were meant to be slim and healthy. Don't let old excuses, old prejudices or old friends cheat you of that.

· *ATTITUDE ADJUSTING* ·

Before you began to lose weight, I explained to you that you would find dieting very difficult if you ate for all the wrong reasons. Have you licked those attitudes for good, or will you still find yourself running to food for comfort?

Perhaps the most demoralizing thing in the world is to deliberately overeat, knowing while you do it that you don't need the food and that it will make you fat. Binge . . . guilt . . . more binges . . . more guilt. Once back on that downward spiral, you'll find it very hard to break out.

So I'm going to tell you one thing that you're probably not going to like very much but needs to be said: your compulsive need to overeat is a symptom of discontent — worry, frustration, boredom, restriction and so on. Food isn't the basic problem and you must look beyond that in order to cure your weight problem for good.

You can do this in three stages.

First, find a substitute crutch. It shouldn't be alcohol, drugs or tobacco, of course. It could be a friend or neighbour, a parent, a child, a pen-pal, a counsellor, a Samaritan even. A biscuit is no substitute for a good listener or some good advice.

Second, every single time you feel like turning to food as a substitute for any other aspect of life, get in the habit of doing something positive. A binge lowers your self-esteem and in the long run makes your problems seem worse. Positive action of almost any kind will *raise* your self-esteem and get you on an upward spiral instead. What is a positive action? Anything at all that gives pleasure, help, enjoyment or enlightenment to you — or to anyone else. It could be anything from reading a book or magazine to visiting an elderly neighbour, to taking up a hobby, tidying out neglected cupboards or joining an evening class. Do it once; you'll see I'm right. Do it several times, you're winning. From small positive actions, it's but a small step to stage three.

Third, set to work on those major areas of discontent in your life, or whatever it is about yourself that is really bugging you. Go on – don't accept life; really think about what's wrong. Don't be frightened of life and all it has to offer. You slimmed, so you can do anything. That should be your attitude. Don't be paralysed by fear of failure. That was the old you. The new you works out what is wrong, what you can do about it, and if you think you can't do anything, why not?

All this will take more nerve and more effort than overeating. But at the end of the day, food *is* only food.

Life is more than just a jam doughnut.

And you, too, deserve your share.

· A SUMMARY OF WHAT YOU'VE READ IN CHAPTER 10 ·

· Staying slim is even more important than getting slim.

· You *don't* have to 'eat like a rabbit' for the rest of your life in order to stay slim.

· You *do* have to eat a little less than you did when you were overweight.

· People's calorie needs vary widely; don't compare yourself with others.

· Gradually build up the amount of food you eat after dieting gradually until you discover your own maintenance level.

· Keep a regular eye on the scales to ensure you never gain more than a very few pounds.

· Accept food for what it is, and accept yourself as a slim person – for life!

11 · JUNK FOOD FOR KIDS

At teatime every day of the year throughout the country, millions of mums serve beefburger and chips or fish fingers and chips to their appreciative children — and feel deeply, uncontrollably guilty for doing so.

Kids love all the things that we've been led to believe are 'bad' for them, and most would rather starve than eat brown rice, broccoli or boiled fish. No wonder that even the most well-intentioned of parents give up the fight to provide their children with a 'healthier' diet. What all parents want is for their children to be healthy, strong, fit and slim. But they also — very badly — want them to enjoy their food.

In this chapter, I aim to prove that the two are compatible, and that many of your worries about your children's diet are unfounded.

· CHILDREN'S NUTRITIONAL REQUIREMENTS* ·

Although there are broad similarities between what children need and what adults need for good health, there are also some important differences.

You'll have read in Chapter 2 (refresh your memory now!) about a good adult diet. Here are the main differences when it comes to your children:

*Age five and over.

TABLE 8

CHILDREN'S NUTRIENT NEEDS – DAILY*

Age	Calories	Protein (g)	Calcium (mg)	Iron (mg)	Vitamin C (mg)
Boys					
5–6	1,740	43	600	10	20
7–8	1,980	49	600	10	20
9–11	2,280	56	700	12	25
12–14	2,640	66	700	12	25
15–17	2,880	72	600	12	30
Comparison with an adult male, 35–64, moderately active	2,750	69	500	10	30
Girls					
5–6	1,680	42	600	10	20
7–8	1,900	48	600	10	20
9–11	2,050	51	700	12	25
12–14	2,150	53	700	12	25
15–17	2,150	53	600	12	30
Comparison with an adult female, 18–54, most occupations	2,150	54	500	12	30

*Figures from Ministry of Agriculture's *Manual of Nutrition* (HMSO).

• Children's protein needs in relation to their size are higher than an adults' (see Table 8). An average ten-year-old boy needs as much as, or even a little more than, most women, and a ten-year-old girl needs almost as much.

• Children of *all* ages need more calcium than all adults, apart from women who are pregnant or breastfeeding. Their need for calcium is so high because they are forming bones and teeth. Need peaks at adolescence, when the UK recommended daily amount is 700 mg (see Table 8). To help convert the calcium to strong bone, children also need sufficient vitamin D. In summer enough is supplied by sunlight on skin but in winter a daily 10 ug is recommended. (Doses higher than 50 ug can be dangerous, though.)

• Iron needs are high in relation to size. A six-year-old child needs as much iron as an adult male, and by the time she's ten, a girl needs more than a man (see Table 8).

• A high-fibre diet is not necessarily a good idea unless your child has constipation or tends towards being overweight. Because children's nutrient needs are high in relation to the size of their digestive systems and stomachs, a very high-bulk diet may mean they simply cannot eat enough to satisfy those requirements.

• And lastly, children's calorie needs are high in relation to their size. By the time a boy is seven or eight, he may be needing as many calories as his mother, for example (see Table 8). This means they need plenty of carbohydrate-rich foods to supply that energy.

Children also need all the other nutrients that adults need: enough vitamin C and all the other trace elements, in correspondingly smaller amounts.

How important is it to limit the amount of fat, sugar and salt in your child's diet?

Although our taste in food usually changes as we grow older, the diet we eat as children plays a large part in deciding what we eat as adults. Although young children rarely suffer from the type of heart disease that adults get or have high blood pressure, and they certainly don't succumb to mid-life-onset diabetes, what your children eat at ten years old will give them habits that last a lifetime. So it is important that the habits learnt are good ones. It's wise that they should learn to enjoy a diet that doesn't contain too much animal fat; that they should not get into the habit of eating too much high-salt food, or of adding salt to food at the table; and, for the sake of their future waistline and good health as well as the immediate well-being of their teeth, that they should, perhaps most important of all, not develop an obsessive liking for very sweet, sugary foods.

So how does a 'junk food' diet fit in with these rather exacting nutritional requirements? In many respects, quite well. In fact, parents who are over-enthusiastic in their attempts to give their children a healthy diet may be doing more harm than good.

Let's look again at children's special needs in the context of a 'junk food' diet.

Plenty of calories

The fact that some 'junk food' can be fattening is of relevance only if your child is putting on too much weight. But for most parents, the problem is more likely to be one of finding enough food to give a ravenous child who never seems to put on an ounce! The best way to supply your children with calories is to give them 'high-density' foods like cakes, biscuits, meat and cheese. Fat is the highest-density food there is, so you can include a sensible amount of butter or margarine and fried foods in a slim child's diet without feeling guilty. Many of the so-called 'junk' foods aimed specifically at kids – fish fingers, burgers, goujons, grilled or baked – are not at all high in fat, and most children have a natural aversion to eating fat that's been left on cooked meat – shoulder of lamb, or bacon, for instance. So as long as you apply all the rules and guidelines that appeared in the adult Junk Food Diet regarding fat to your child's diet too, you won't need to worry.

So don't feel guilty about those chips – a well-cooked plateful supplies not only calories for a hungry growing child but also some valuable vitamin C and some protein. What you *don't* want to do when your children are hungry is give them a packet of sweets. Sweet foods will satisfy hunger only for a short time; they contain no 'goodness' and will give the wrong idea about sensible eating. More about sweet foods later though.

Plenty of protein

Many 'junk' foods are a good source of low-fat protein – all of those based on lean beef, poultry and fish are good additions to your child's diet. Eggs, sausages (especially the low-fat kinds), frankfurters, baked beans are too. And most of the carbohydrate-rich foods like potatoes and bread contain reasonable amounts of protein. Some of these foods have a medium or high added-salt content, so if you're watching salt in your child's diet, it's worth limiting the higher-salt items (see Table 9) to occasional meals, and make sure never to let your child add salt to meals at the table.

TABLE 9
HIGH-SALT FOODS
(EXCLUDING REDUCED-SALT VERSIONS, WHICH WILL BE CLEARLY LABELLED)

All the foods below have a high salt content, but the ones at the top have most.

Yeast extract	Tomato ketchup
Shrimps	Sausages
Olives	Luncheon-meat
Bacon products	Brown sauce
Salami	Corned beef
Sweet pickle	Canned soups, packet soups
Prawns	Beefburgers
Blue cheese	Pork pie
Processed cheese	Canned sardines
Ham	Most other cheeses
Smoked haddock	Crisps
Black pudding	Kippers
Cornflakes	Canned spaghetti

Plenty of calcium

Far and away the best sources of calcium are milk (whole, semi-skimmed and skimmed), yogurt and hard cheeses, all of which provide other valuable nutrients, such as protein, too. A pint of milk a day will give your children their full day's calcium requirement. A small tub of yogurt will provide a third, as will enough cheese for a sandwich.

Although cottage and skimmed-milk soft cheeses are much lower in fat than Cheddar, they have a relatively low calcium content, so I think that the higher-fat Cheddar, cheese spreads and medium-fat cream cheeses are a better bet for children. The only other foods with appreciable amounts of calcium per serving are sardines (if your child eats the bones, which many won't), white bread and leafy green vegetables.

So you begin to see why dairy produce is so valuable for children, especially ones who won't 'eat up their greens'.

If your children aren't keen on 'straight' milk or natural yogurt, it is far better to let them drink a milk shake or a hot chocolate and eat fruit yogurt, or even custard, rice pudding or ice cream, than to see them go short of their calcium.

Plenty of iron

Your child may be one of the few children who adores liver and begs for it – but if he or she does, you're in the minority! Liver and other offal are the best sources of iron, but next best are all the red meats. (That maligned beefburger is looking more like the good guy every minute, isn't it?) Eggs, chips, peas, white bread and fortified breakfast cereals are also good sources. Even chocolate contains iron, and baked beans do too.

So is junk food absolved?

Children who eat cornflakes or Rice Krispies for breakfast, burger and (properly cooked) chips for lunch at school, beans on white toast when they get home, plus a Cheddar cheese and crackers snack later, are certainly not eating what I would call junk food – not by any means. As far as it goes, such a diet goes a long way towards providing them with all the nutrients they need for good health. But where your child's diet is likely to go wrong from here is in two important ways:

First, it may not get the addition of fruit and vegetables that your child needs for the vital vitamins and minerals they supply (especially vitamin C).

It is a very unusual child who isn't faddy about one vegetable or another. Highest on the hate-list is anything green and leafy – cabbage and sprouts, for instance. But don't give up on *all* vegetables because of the refusal of one or two. Your children need vegetables and fruit, and there will always be something they are going to like – or at least eat without too much fuss.

A fairly comprehensive list of the best sources of vitamin C appears on page 41.

Second, the addition of too many sweet and/or fatty and/or salty and/or low-nutrient snacks and extras may turn a perfectly healthy 'junk food' diet into a less healthy one, if you aren't careful. Even worse, if you aren't careful, these low-nutrient snack foods may become so appealing to your children that they begin to replace the higher-quality foods in their diet.

Here are my guidelines on the subject for a child who is slim or within the normal weight range for his or her height. There are different guidelines for overweight children towards the end of the chapter.

• If your child has a big appetite get into the habit of satisfying his or her hunger with a bread snack or nut and fruit snacks. If the diet is not, otherwise, very high in salt, there is nothing wrong with the occasional packet of crisps – in fact, the new-style, jacket potato crisps cooked in oil with not too much added salt are a nutritious snack and a reasonable addition to a lunchbox.

• If your child likes cakes and/or biscuits, give him or her the lower-sugar kinds which do contain various nutrients – fruit cake or carrot cake, for example, rather than jam sponge, and digestive or oat cookies rather than sugar-icing-coated cookies.

• Yogurts, custards and all milk-based puddings are a better bet for children than pavlovas and treacle sponges, if you want to give your child a dessert. Fruit-based puddings are best of all.

• If your child asks for sweets, limit them to a definite time — say, a packet at weekends only, or a few sweets at night after tea.

• Sweets usually contain nothing but sugar, water, colourings and flavourings, and add nothing whatsoever to the goodness of your child's diet. Boiled sweets, chews, jelly sweets, wine gums, toffees and any sweet, gooey, sticky foods are the ones which are most likely to leave the deposits on your child's teeth which start the process that leads to dental decay.

• Try to give sugary foods as part of a meal rather than on their own, and remember that the longer the sweet food is in contact with your child's teeth, the more potential damage it can do, so it is better to give children a bar or a sweet item that they can eat straight away rather than, say, a packet of pastilles that they may suck for hours.

• Get your child into the habit of cleaning his or her teeth after every meal and/or after every time he or she has eaten a sweet item. As children can't (or don't) clean their teeth at school, it is best not to include high-sugar items in your child's lunchbox.

• Don't replace nutritious drinks such as fruit juice and milk with low-nutrient or no-nutrient drinks like cola and squashes. Sugary drinks are similar to sweets in that they often contain nothing but sugar, water and colourings and flavourings, so use them only occasionally. The cheapest drink to quench thirst is water!

• Don't allow your child to eat sweets, chocolate, popcorn and the like instead of a meal.

• If your child doesn't have a sweet tooth, don't encourage one to develop with regular bribes or presents of sweets and chocolate.

Limit – or ban?

The reason I say sweet foods and snacks should be limited in your child's diet rather than completely banned is simple: if there is one way to ensure that children want something, it is to tell them they can't have it. Add to that the natural fascination of something that is forbidden and you have children who will, once they're of school age, find a supply of sweets, chocolate or whatever come what may, despite your best efforts. That way you have no control.

However, if we offer your children a sensible compromise – the occasional item – they will be less concerned about it. In other words, those sweet treats and extras should be limited in your child's diet in just the same way they are on the adult Junk Food Diet and maintenance plan.

By doing this, you will be getting your children used to the idea of balance, variety and moderation in their diet, an idea that will do them nothing but good all their life.

How do you know you're helping them to get the balance right? If they're not overweight, if they're in good health with a full set of teeth and regular dental check-ups, you're doing okay.

· JUNK FOOD AND ALLERGIES ·

Because additive-knocking is the current national pastime, it's little wonder that more and more parents are asking, 'Is it the additives?' when their child has a rash, is sick, has a runny nose, is lethargic or hyperactive (surely the most over-used word of the decade).

The additives debate is never more fierce than when it concerns our kids. Let me say straight away that no one is

TABLE 10

TRAFFIC LIGHT GUIDE TO KID'S 'JUNK' FOOD*

	Food type	Your attitude should be
GREEN	Children's favourite meals: beefburgers, fish fingers, chicken goujons, turkey burgers, fried eggs, pizzas, hot dogs, etc.	Don't feel guilty if your child enjoys these foods. If you ring the changes and add vegetables and/or fruit to the meal, they are fine. Follow the 'fat guidelines' above.
	Chips	If properly cooked, a good source of energy, protein and vitamin C. But don't forget alternatives, like baked potatoes or even instant mash now and then!
	White bread	An excellent choice for most children – white contains more calcium than wholemeal bread. For extra fibre, soft grain white is the ideal choice.
	Baked beans	Good food – the low-sugar, low-salt kind are even better.
AMBER	Puddings and desserts	Yogurts, milk puddings, ice cream, custard and instant whips all supply calcium. Fruit with

		calcium-rich accompaniment is a good pudding for kids, but other puds are best kept as occasional happenings.
	Snacks – crisps, salted peanuts	Fine in reasonable quantities for the hungry child, but think about the salt content; choose low-salt versions if possible.
	Cake, biscuits, chocolate	Think of them as occasional items.
RED	Sweets and fizzy drinks	High-sugar, low nutrient foods. Limit severely.

arguing the fact that some children are allergic to some additives. The most common food additive to cause allergy in recent years has been the yellow food dye, tartrazine (E102). Nowadays it's hard to find a food that contains tartrazine – manufacturers wisely decided to find alternatives – but it is the food dye group as a whole that appears to cause the most frequent allergy problems.

That said, for every child who is genuinely allergic to an additive, there are thousands who are not. In the 1987 Ministry of Agriculture-sponsored High Wycombe food additives trials, only one child out of 1,376 respondents (of all ages) who thought they had food additive intolerance was found to be genuinely allergic to an additive (an azo dye). And no evidence at all was found to support the theory that hyperactivity and other behaviour problems are directly caused by food additives; nor has there been proof from any other trials, to my knowledge.

Ironically, it is by no means the case that food additives are the biggest cause of allergic reactions – far from it. The most common triggers of allergic reactions are wheat, milk, eggs, shellfish, strawberries and nuts – all foods that we regard as 'healthy' and 'natural'. Proven allergies to food additives come after this list.

It is estimated that up to one in twenty of the population may be allergic to a greater or lesser degree to one food or another. The most common symptoms are tingling or itchy skin, nettle rash, asthma, nausea and diarrhoea.

If you think your child may be allergic to a food or a food additive, talk to your doctor, who may suggest an elimination programme to confirm the allergy or other suitable treatment. However, bearing in mind the trial I quoted earlier in the chapter, don't be surprised if the symptoms turn out to be not the result of a food additive allergy at all.

Food additives that appear to cause the most frequent reactions in children are E102, E104, 107, E110, E120, E122, E123, E124, E127, 128, E132, E133, E150, E151, 154, 155, E210, E211, E220, E250, E320, E321, 621.

Don't forget that all additives in food on sale for human consumption in this country have been approved by the government after what they consider to be adequate tests. However, if you are one of the many parents who still prefer to cut down on additives 'to be on the safe side', it is becoming an easier and easier task to do so.

First, the manufacturers are voluntarily removing many unnecessary additives from their products, especially artificial colourings (those dyes that cause most of the allergy problems that do occur) and flavourings which are really only there for cosmetic purposes. And second, because by law the manufacturer has to include a list of ingredients including additives on the packaging of all but a very few foods, it is a fairly easy matter to check the packets at the supermarket for the additives you want to avoid. This is particularly useful if there is just one you need to cut out.

If you want further reading on the subject of additives I can't do better than recommend *E for Additives* by Maurice Hanssen (published by Thorsons), which is the accepted additives Bible.

· JUNK FOOD, PERSONALITY AND ABILITY ·

I frequently hear parents discussing whether their children's bad temper, mood swings, laziness, tendency to pinch money from the housekeeping jar – or a thousand and one other slight variations on normal childhood behaviour – is due in some way to lack of the right food in their diet.

And the 'breakthrough discovery' last year that schoolchildren became brainier when given vitamin and mineral supplements added plenty of fuel to this fire. It's a tempting thought: supplement your child's diet with a couple of pills a day and in place of a sullen, awkward, (typical?) teenager you'll find a bright, well-mannered genius.

However, wait a minute. Different government-sponsored trials have shown that only a small minority of British schoolchildren actually do have a diet that, according to its own nutrient tables, are lacking in any nutrients at all. (Yes, really. You see, even without my help you weren't doing too badly at feeding your child, were you?)

As you will remember if you read Chapter 2, giving a

person extra vitamins or minerals when they already have enough, is a total waste of time. Also, a more recent trial found no link between schoolchildren's intelligence and vitamin supplements.

So the only sensible conclusion I can come to is this: if you give your children a varied diet, even one that includes lots of burgers and chips galore, it is *highly unlikely* that diet will be to blame if they perform poorly at school or if they're not quite the perfect children you think they ought to be.

The Junk Food for Kids principles will give your children all they need in the way of nutrients, including vitamins and minerals, and if they are in normal health and eating well, I don't see any point at all in giving them supplements (especially as they are so costly) in the vague hope that they'll turn into the amicable academic you always knew they were!

If they are getting a poor diet – say, your child really will eat only crisps and bananas, or bread and Marmite; or is a really faddy eater with a poor appetite; or is or has been ill – then see your doctor, who will give you whatever advice you need and will probably recommend a suitable supplement – on prescription.

And I strongly advise you *not* to rely on supplements for your child instead of a good diet, and *not* to give your child high doses of any one vitamin or mineral, because, as we saw in Chapter 2, megadoses *can* be dangerous.

· OVERWEIGHT CHILDREN ·

Surprisingly, perhaps, only 2 per cent of boys and 4 per cent of girls up to the age of eleven are truly overweight –

that is, more than 20 per cent over the average weight for a child of their sex and height.

Is your child overweight? Let's find out.

The height/weight chart opposite (Table 11) will give you a fair guide as to what your child's weight should be, but before you look at it, bear in mind the following:

· The heights given for the ages are average for that age. But if your child is smaller or taller than the height listed for his or her age, then read the correct weight from height not age. For girls taller than 5 ft 4 in and boys taller than 5 ft 9 in, check the adult chart on page 86–7.

· Remember that two children of the same age and height will vary in weight and still both be within an acceptable range.

· Use the charts in conjunction with your own common sense. For instance, do your children *look* overweight? Are they much heavier than all the other children in their class? How do they look without clothes on: are they flabby? Do you find it hard to get clothes to fit them: for example, are the clothes the right length but always too tight? You can probably tell more by using these visual methods than by using the chart, which *is only a guide*.

Approximately 10 per cent either side of the average weights given can be described as normal. But if your child reaches, or exceeds, the 20 per cent upper limit given on the right-hand side of the chart, it is almost certain that he or she is overweight. Any weight between 10 per cent above normal and 20 per cent above normal is perhaps a case of being mildly overweight – and a warning for you to watch and make sure your child doesn't reach the 20 per cent limit. Use the points above to help you make a sensible decision.

TABLE 11

HEIGHT/WEIGHT CHART FOR CHILDREN
Average weight for girls*

Age	Height	Average weight	10% above	20% above
5	42 in	40 lb	44 lb	48 lb
	106 cm	18·25 kg	20 kg	22 kg
6	45 in	45 lb	49·5 lb	54 lb
	114 cm	20·5 kg	22·5 kg	24·5 kg
7	47 in	50 lb	55 lb	60 lb
	120 cm	22·75 kg	25 kg	27·25 kg
8	49 in	55 lb	60·5 lb	66 lb
	124 cm	25 kg	27·5 kg	30 kg
9	51 in	62 lb	68·25 lb	74·5 lb
	130 cm	28·25 kg	31 kg	34 kg
10	54 in	68 lb	74·75 lb	81·5 lb
	137 cm	31 kg	34 kg	37·25 kg
11	56 in	76 lb	83·5 lb	91·25 lb
	142 cm	34·5 kg	38 kg	41·5 kg
12	58 in	89 lb	98 lb	107 lb
	147 cm	40·5 kg	44·5 kg	48·5 kg
13	62 in	104 lb	114·5 lb	125 lb
	157 cm	47·25 kg	52 kg	57 kg
14	63 in	115 lb	126.5 lb	138 lb
	160 cm	52·25 kg	57·5 kg	63 kg
15	64 in	121 lb	133 lb	145 lb
	163 cm	57 kg	63 kg	68 kg
16	64 in	125 lb	137 lb	150 lb
	163 cm	57 kg	63 kg	68 kg
17	64 in	126 lb	138 lb	151 lb
	163 cm	57·5 kg	63·25 kg	69 kg

* (For girls 18 +, see adult chart on page 86).

TABLE 11
HEIGHT/WEIGHT CHART FOR CHILDREN
Average weight for boys*

Age	Height	Average weight	10% above	20% above
5	43 in	41 lb	45 lb	49·5 lb
	109 cm	18·5 kg	20·5 kg	22·5 kg
6	45 in	46 lb	50·5 lb	55·25 lb
	114 cm	21 kg	23 kg	25 kg
7	48 in	50 lb	55 lb	60 lb
	122 cm	22·75 kg	25 kg	27·25 kg
8	50 in	55 lb	60·5 lb	66 lb
	127 cm	25 kg	27·5 kg	30 kg
9	52 in	62 lb	68·25 lb	74·5 lb
	132 cm	28·25 kg	31 kg	34 kg
10	54 in	68 lb	74·75 lb	81·5 lb
	137 cm	31 kg	34 kg	37·25 kg
11	56 in	74 lb	81·5 lb	89 lb
	142 cm	33·5 kg	37 kg	40·5 kg
12	58 in	81 lb	89 lb	97 lb
	147 cm	37 kg	40·5 kg	44 kg
13	60 in	91 lb	100 lb	109 lb
	152 cm	41·5 kg	45·5 kg	49·5 kg
14	63 in	106 lb	117 lb	127 lb
	160 cm	48 kg	53 kg	58 kg
15	66 in	122 lb	134 lb	146 lb
	167 cm	55·5 kg	61 kg	66·5 kg
16	68 in	133 lb	146 lb	160 lb
	173 cm	60·5 kg	66·5 kg	73 kg
17	69 in	136 lb	150 lb	163 lb
	175 cm	62 kg	68 kg	74 kg
18	69 in	140 lb	154 lb	168 lb
	175 cm	64 kg	70 kg	76·5 kg

* (For boys 19 +, see adult chart on page 87).

If you have come to the conclusion that yes, your child *is* overweight, what should you do?

Don't impose a very strict diet. If he or she is mildly overweight — say, just over the 10 per cent above average weight for the height (for example, if a girl is 3 ft 11 in tall and weighs 56 lb she could *perhaps* do with being a few pounds less. But rather than put her on an active slimming diet, it is probably better to put her on a 'containing' diet — one which will keep her the same weight for the next few months so that eventually she will gain enough height to slim down naturally. Most children grow an average of 2–3 inches a year, which should result, depending upon her age, in a surplus of up to half a stone being 'lost' in this way.

If, however, she is 20 per cent plus overweight (60 lb or more), you could put her on a gradual slimming diet.

What you *don't* want to do is totally ignore her weight problem and hope that it will disappear of its own accord, without you having to keep any kind of eye on what she eats. Your child *needs* your help in order to slim down. Overeating, in childhood as in adulthood, is a habit that can be hard to break.

· GETTING THE WEIGHT OFF ·

I am not going to give you a set low-calorie diet for your child, because calorie counting depends so much on age, height, the scale of problem and other factors. Also, if children are put 'on a diet' and know it, they are more likely to rebel, or cheat, or get bored.

If you decide to devise your own diet, I'd strongly advise you not to put him or her on one that is less than 500 calories a day below the average calorie requirement for a child of that sex and age (see the chart on page 226), with an absolute minimum calorie level for any child of 1,250. I would also advise that any weight loss above 1 lb a week for a child up to 5 ft tall, and any loss above 2 lb a week for a child over 5 ft tall, is too high. It would also make sense for you to see a doctor if you think your child is seriously overweight.

So how do you achieve that weight loss without a diet as such?

This is what you do. Go back to the Traffic Light Guide to Junk Food for your Kids (see pages 235–6).

First, you cut back on all the RED foods in your child's diet – the sugary things that aren't giving any of the nutrients needed for health. If there has been a lot of this kind of item, you may have to cut back gradually, and replace some of them with more nutritious foods – swop a bag of sweets for a small slice of fruit cake, for instance. You could also swop sugary colas and drinks for the calorie-free kind made with artificial sweeteners, although long-term it's best to get your child used to water or fruit juice as a drink.

At the same time, you can swop whole milk for skimmed milk, and butter in sandwiches, and so on, for low-fat spread. These are changes that will probably not even be noticed. If your child takes sugar in tea or coffee, gradually reduce the amount you put in. If you reduce it almost grain by grain, it won't be noticed (I promise!).

After a couple of weeks on this plan, weigh your child. If any weight has been lost – say, a pound or two – that could be enough on its own. If no weight has been lost – perhaps because there weren't many sweets in the diet anyway – move on to the next step.

This is to replace the AMBER items on the chart with lower-calorie ones, or to cut them out altogether. For example, you could replace a large slice of chocolate cake with a small slice of fruit cake, or three chocolate biscuits with two plain ones. You could replace a fruit pie and cream dessert with a yogurt and fruit fool. Or a jam sponge and custard with stewed fruit and custard. Whatever you do, don't apologize when you hand over any of these 'swops'. If you don't mention the reason, the child will never get a chance to feel hard done by.

Get scales out again in a couple of weeks. If a pound or two has been lost, continue on the same lines. I expect most children will be losing a little weight by this time. If not, or if the weight loss is marginal, proceed as follows.

Substitute all cake, biscuits and puddings for fresh fruit desserts or diet yogurts – but allow one small treat a day, maximum 150 calories. Cut down on the amount of chips, or swop them most of the time with boiled potato or baked potato, and if your child's been having large portions of his main meal for his age, cut down on the amount of food on the plate. You won't save all that many calories by cutting down on the amount of vegetables (apart from fried ones), and in any case they help you to fill up, so I'd cut down a little on meat, pastry, battered foods, first – perhaps give a little less rice, pasta or potato, and don't bother adding hunks of butter to the plate. Make sure gravy is strained of fat.

Don't cut down on fruit and I wouldn't suggest cutting down on bread drastically, unless your child has literally been getting through half a loaf or more a day.

Talking of which, some children will be overweight because of an obsessive liking for one particular food – crisps, say, or cake, or biscuits, perhaps. Do all you can to get them to cut down on that food: if it's something they eat mostly at home, simply buy less. While freeing them of their obsession for this particular food, don't let them go hungry. Substitute other foods, even if they aren't low-calorie ones. Then, when you have the single-food fetish licked, you can begin the slimming process, using the method outlined above.

It is very hard to slim down a rebellious child, and for that reason it is essential that you keep his or her cooperation all along the line. With most children, this means doing it in the way I've described: slimming them without there ever being a point at which you say, 'Right, you're going on a diet.' To this end, it will help a great deal if all the family make some, or all, of the diet changes I've outlined; if you've been following the Junk Food Diet yourself, you are probably halfway there already.

· PLANNING YOUR CHILD'S MENU ·

Build up a healthy diet for your child with the help of the meal ideas and tips that follow.

No busy parent has the time to be a nutritionist. A large part of planning a good diet is instinctive. The most important rule, perhaps, is to vary your family's meals so that they don't have the same food too often (the exception, of course, being staples such as bread and potatoes, which can be eaten every day and without which we would find providing meals very hard). A fairly simple way of ensuring your child gets all the nutrients necessary for good health is to follow the 'food group' principle.

Give *two* servings a day from Group 1, the foods rich in protein. These are lean meat, offal, poultry, fish, eggs, beans, nuts and pulses.

Give *three* servings a day or more from Group 2, the foods rich in carbohydrate. These are potatoes, bread, rice, pasta and breakfast cereals.

Give *three* servings a day from Group 3, the calcium-rich foods. These are milk, cheese and yogurt.

Give *three* servings a day or more from Group 4, the

vitamin- and mineral-rich foods. These are fruit and vegetables.

This table rather over-simplifies food, because most of the foods overlap into other groups: for example, the Group 2 foods also contain protein, the Group 3 foods are good sources of protein, and all the foods mentioned, not just fruit and vegetables, contain vitamins and minerals. However, it is a very good guide to follow.

Another simple way to ensure reasonable nutrition is to make sure that at every meal your child has a protein-rich food, a carbohydrate-rich food, and a fruit or vegetable, plus a pint of milk a day.

A meal doesn't have to be a traditional 'meat and two veg' type to be nutritious: you could get the right mix from a plate of beans (protein) on toast (carbohydrate) plus a piece of fresh fruit.

And the meal doesn't have to be cooked either: a Ploughman's Lunch with a tomato or two is just as nutritious as a roast meal.

Here are some more tips that will help you plan your children's daily menu:

• Give them a breakfast every day. You may not eat, or need, breakfast, but a breakfast will ensure that your children get a percentage of the nutrients they need, and they may not get another chance to eat until lunchtime, which isn't a good idea. The alternative is that they will feel ravenous by morning breaktime and, more than likely, eat a sugary snack instead of something more nutritious.

• Give them a packed lunch if possible, so that you can have control over what they eat. The second-best idea is for them to buy a school meal — even if there is a choice, most of the alternatives will be reasonably high on nutrients. The worst option is for your children to go outside the school and buy what they like. Research shows that they are then most likely to get a very unbalanced meal — a bag of chips, for instance, or even nothing at all.

• Remember, variety and balance are the key. The wider your choice of foods, the more likely your children are to get all they need for health.

12 · THE JUNK FOOD DIET RECIPES

You don't need to be a brilliant cook, or even an experienced one, to whip up the simple recipes that follow. And you certainly don't need a lot of spare time. So, although you can follow the Junk Food Diet perfectly well without trying even one of these dishes, it's well worth giving some of them a go. They will add even more variety to your diet and are an added precaution against boredom!

Each recipe had to pass a very stringent test before I allowed it to be included! It had to fulfil at least six out of seven of the following criteria:

- Easy to shop for, prepare and cook.
- Quick to prepare and cook. A few recipes have a longish cooking time, but you can be doing something else while the cooking's in progress, so that isn't necessarily a minus point.
- More-ish. The bland and the dull have been banished. I know what your tastebuds like.
- Not depressingly obvious 'slimmer's fare'. I love meals that sound fattening when in fact they're not! And I don't see the point of cooking depressing-sounding dishes like 'Dieter's fish and celery casserole'. I thought you would agree with me, which is why my recipes include such glorious meals as chilli con carne, lasagne, moussaka and spaghetti Bolognese!
- Suitable for everyone. The recipes serve four, two or one, depending upon which is most suitable for that particular dish. However, many of the family meals can

quite easily be cooked in smaller quantities: just divide the ingredients accordingly.

    • No hard-to-find ingredients, or unfamiliar ones. Most of us are familiar with paprika and soured cream by now, and that's about as far as you'll need to go.

    • Inexpensive. I've tried hard not to major on lobster, fruits out of season or smoked salmon. Most of the meals will fit in well with your food budget. One or two are more special, included deliberately in the hope that you'll be wanting a celebration meal now and then — celebrating your weight loss, I expect.

The recipes can be used in two ways: either as part of your Junk Food Diet, in which case you'll find the number of the page(s) where the recipe appears at the top of each recipe. Calories given are per portion *for the recipe only*. Any suggested accompaniments or any foods that may accompany the dish within the diets are not included, which is why, for instance, a 400-calorie recipe may be included in the 500-calorie meal lists in the Pick Your Own Plan.

You can also use the recipes on your maintenance plan (see Chapter 10) as and when you wish.

To prove that some of the recipes aren't as 'bad for you' as they sound, I've given each one a star-rated nutritional breakdown covering fat, fibre, protein, iron, calcium and vitamin C. For each of these, ★★★ means high, ★★ means medium and ★ means low. In the case of fat, 'high' means over 20 g per portion, but don't forget that much of the fat in the recipes is mono- and polyunsaturated (the 'good for you' kinds).

Remember, with all recipes it is best to use the freshest ingredients you can find, and you should weigh and measure ingredients carefully.

· SAUCES ·

Cheese sauce (see pages 107, 124, 135, 171, 254, 265)

SERVES 4
Calories per portion: 155
Preparation and cooking time: 10 minutes
Fat ★ Fibre ★ Protein ★★★ Iron ★ Calcium ★★★ Vitamin C ★

½ oz (15 g) butter
1 tablespoon flour
1 pint (600 ml) skimmed milk
4 oz (115 g) Shape or Tendale Cheddar-style cheese, grated
Pinch salt and pepper

Melt the butter in a saucepan over medium heat. Shake in the flour and continue cooking for a minute, stirring. Gradually add the milk, stirring to avoid lumps. Add the cheese and stir until blended; add salt and pepper to taste.
NOTE: Make Parsley Sauce, at only 90 calories a portion, by omitting the cheese and adding 2 tablespoons chopped fresh parsley.

Tomato sauce (see pages 259, 260, 272)

SERVES 4
Calories per portion: 80
Preparation and cooking time: 20 minutes
Fat ★ Fibre ★ Protein ★ Iron ★★ Calcium ★ Vitamin C ★★★

1 Spanish onion, very finely chopped
1 × 15 oz (425 g) can chopped tomatoes
1 tablespoon tomato purée
1 in garlic purée (optional)
2 tablespoons olive or corn oil
1 teaspoon dried oregano or parsley

Heat the oil in a non-stick pan, then add the onions and cook over a medium heat until transparent and soft. Add the rest of the ingredients and simmer for about 15 minutes, until you have a thick sauce. This should be salty enough, but you can add a little if you must! For a smoother sauce, put through blender.

Barbecue sauce (see pages 123, 134, 264)

SERVES 4
Calories per portion: 55
Preparation and cooking time: 10 minutes
Fat ★ Fibre ★ Protein ★ Iron ★ Calcium ★ Vitamin C ★

1 tablespoon olive or corn oil
1 tablespoon red wine vinegar (malt vinegar will do)
1 tablespoon clear honey
1 heaped tablespoon tomato purée
2 tablespoons soy sauce
1 dessertspoon gravy mix powder
1 teaspoon mixed herbs
Pinch cayenne pepper
4 tablespoons water
$\frac{1}{2}$ in garlic purée

Blend all the ingredients thoroughly in a bowl, then bring to boil in a small saucepan and simmer for a few minutes until you have a rich, coating sauce. (Even if you think you don't like garlic, do try the garlic purée in this recipe!)

· BREAD SNACKS ·

Chicken and Mushroom Pitta (see page 160)

SERVES 2
Calories per portion: 350
Preparation and cooking time: 5 minutes
Fat ★★ Fibre ★★ Protein ★★★ Iron ★★ Calcium ★ Vitamin C ★

1 × 7½ oz (213 g) can sliced mushrooms in cream sauce
2 pittas
4 oz (115 g) cooked chicken meat, diced
½ teaspoon paprika
Chopped parsley to garnish

Heat the mushrooms in a small pan and warm the pittas
(optional). Add the chicken and paprika to the mushrooms
and mix well. Halve the pittas and fill them with the
mushroom mixture. Add parsley garnish (optional).

Tuna Pitta (see page 160)

SERVES 2
Calories per portion: 350
Preparation time: 5 minutes
Fat ★ Fibre ★★ Protein ★★★ Iron ★★ Calcium ★★ Vitamin
C ★★★

2 pittas
1 × 6½ oz (185 g) can John West Tuna in Barbecue Sauce
2 tomatoes, roughly chopped
4 spring onions, chopped
1 in cucumber, chopped

Warm the pittas (optional). Mix all ingredients together
and divide between the split and opened pittas.

Pizza Toasts (see pages 119, 131, 157, 159)

SERVES 2
Calories per portion: 300
Preparation and cooking time: 10 minutes
Fat ★ Fibre ★★ Protein ★★★ Iron ★★ Calcium ★★★
Vitamin C ★★★

2 × 2 oz (55 g) slices bread (from a round loaf if possible)
A little low-fat spread
1 small onion, finely chopped
1 × 7 oz (200 g) can of chopped tomatoes, drained
2 oz (55 g) sliced mushrooms, or red pepper
4 oz (115 g) reduced-fat Cheddar-style cheese, grated
Green olive slices to garnish (optional)
Toast the bread and spread with a little low-fat spread. Mix together the onion, tomatoes and mushrooms. Spread half the cheese on the bread, followed by the tomato mixture and then the rest of the cheese. Pop under grill until the cheese is melted and golden.

· EGG AND CHEESE MEALS ·

Saucy Baked Eggs (see page 154)

SERVES 4
Calories per portion: 350
Preparation and cooking time: 30 minutes
Fat ★★★ Fibre ★ Protein ★★★ Iron ★★ Calcium ★★★
Vitamin C ★

1 pint (600 ml) Cheese Sauce (see recipe page 251)
2 tablespoons corn oil
12 oz (340 g) mushrooms, sliced

4 size-3 eggs
2 oz (55 g) reduced-fat Cheddar-style cheese, grated

Make up the Cheese Sauce as in recipe and keep warm. Heat the oil in a frying-pan and fry the mushrooms over a high heat, stirring all the time, until just cooked but still crisp. Spread them over the bottom of an ovenproof dish. Break the eggs carefully on top of the mushrooms, keeping them separate. Pour over the cheese sauce and top with the grated cheese. Bake at 180°C, Gas Mark 4, for about 15 minutes or until eggs are just set, and serve.

Piperade (see pages 152, 157)

SERVES 2
Calories per portion: 200
Preparation and cooking time: 10 minutes
Fat ★★ Fibre ★ Protein ★★ Iron ★★ Calcium ★★ Vitamin C ★★★

½ oz (15 g) butter
3 size-3 eggs
2 fresh tomatoes or 2 well-drained canned ones, chopped
4 oz (115 g) green and/or red pepper, fresh or frozen, sliced
1 medium onion, finely chopped
2 tablespoons skimmed milk
Little salt and pepper

Melt the butter in a non-stick frying-pan and stir-fry the vegetables for a few minutes until soft. Beat the eggs, milk and seasoning in a bowl and pour into the pan. Cook over a low heat, stirring, until eggs are scrambled.

Spanish Omelette (see pages 117, 128, 153, 164)

SERVES 2
Calories per portion: 300
Preparation and cooking time: 10 minutes
Fat ★★★ Fibre ★ Protein ★★ Iron ★★ Calcium ★★ Vitamin C ★★

1 medium Spanish onion, thinly sliced
½ oz (15 g) butter
2 teaspoons corn oil
6 oz (170 g) boiled potatoes, sliced
3 size-3 eggs
2 tablespoons skimmed milk
A few chopped chives, fresh or dried
Salt and pepper to taste

Melt the butter and oil in a non-stick frying-pan and fry the onion and potatoes until golden. Beat the eggs with the milk, seasoning and chives and pour over the vegetables in the pan. Cook over a medium heat until eggs are set. If you like you can brown the top under a grill. Cut the omelette in half, slide out carefully and serve.

Egg and Potato Pie (see pages 154, 161)

SERVES 4
Calories per portion: 350
Preparation and cooking time: 45 minutes
Fat ★★ Fibre ★ Protein ★★★ Iron ★★ Calcium ★★★
Vitamin C ★★★

1 lb (450 g) potatoes, boiled and sliced
4 tomatoes, sliced
6 oz (175 g) reduced-fat Cheddar-style cheese, grated
4 size-3 eggs

1 pint (600 ml) skimmed milk
A little salt and pepper

Brush a 3-pint (1·7 l) pie dish with a little low-fat spread and layer the potatoes, tomatoes and cheese in it, finishing with a layer of cheese. Beat the eggs, milk and seasoning together and pour over. Bake at 180°C, Gas Mark 4, for 40 minutes, or until set and golden.

· FISH MEALS ·

Tuna Florentino (see pages 113, 124, 136, 166)

SERVES 4
Calories per portion: 350
Preparation and cooking time: 40 minutes
Fat ★★ Fibre ★★ Protein ★★★ Iron ★★ Calcium ★★★
Vitamin C ★★★

1 × 15 oz (425 g) can tomatoes, drained and chopped
1 tablespoon tomato purée
1 oz (30 g) flour
6 oz (175 g) mushrooms, sliced
½ in garlic purée (optional)
1 teaspoon Italian seasoning
Little salt if necessary
2 × 7½ oz (210 g) cans tuna in oil, well drained
4 oz (115 g) chopped spinach, thawed
½ pint (300 ml) natural yogurt
2 teaspoons cornflour
3 oz (75 g) reduced-fat Cheddar-style cheese, grated

In a bowl, mix together the tomatoes, purée, flour, mushrooms, garlic purée, seasoning and tuna (in fairly large chunks). Put mixture in a 2·5 pint (1·4 l) ovenproof dish. Spread spinach over the top. Mix together the yogurt, cornflour, most of the cheese and salt if liked, and spread over top. Sprinkle on rest of cheese. Bake at 200°C, Gas Mark 6, until top is golden.

Fisherman's Pie (see pages 107, 164)
SERVES 4
Calories per portion: 300
Preparation and cooking time: 50 minutes
Fat ★★ Fibre ★★ Protein ★★★ Iron ★★ Calcium ★★
Vitamin C ★★

1 lb (450 g) cod fillet (or any other white fish)
½ pint (300 ml) skimmed milk
½ pint (300 ml) water
Salt and pepper
1 oz (30 g) butter
1 rounded tablespoon flour
2 tablespoons fresh parsley, chopped
2 size-3 eggs, hard-boiled and sliced
1 lb (450 g) made-up weight instant mashed potato

Poach the fish in a pan with the skimmed milk and water and the salt and pepper, until just cooked. Remove fish from pan, reserving liquid. Make a white sauce by melting the butter in a saucepan and adding the flour; cook for a couple of minutes, then gradually add the fish stock, stirring until you have a sauce. Season if necessary, and add the parsley. Place the flaked fish and the eggs in a pie dish and pour the sauce over. Let it settle well, then gently spoon or pipe the potato over the top. Bake at 200°C, Gas Mark 6, for 30 minutes, or until potato is crisp and golden.

Scampi Provençale (see pages 111, 162)

SERVES 4
Calories per portion: 170
Preparation and cooking time: 15 minutes
Fat ★ Fibre ★ Protein ★★ Iron ★★ Calcium ★★ Vitamin C ★★

½ oz (15 g) butter
1 small onion, finely chopped
½ in garlic purée
6 oz (170 g) button mushrooms, sliced
1 tablespoon flour
1 glass (5 fl oz, 150 ml) dry white wine, or equivalent
cooking wine
½ pint (300 ml) fish stock from cube
Salt and pepper to taste
1 tablespoon tomato purée
1 × 7 oz (200 g) can chopped tomatoes
12 oz (340 g) scampi (king prawns), peeled and drained
weight

Melt the butter in a frying-pan and cook the onion over a
medium heat until transparent and soft. Add the garlic
purée, the mushrooms, and stir. Add the flour and stir
again. Add the wine, allow to bubble for a minute, then add
the stock, seasoning, tomato purée, chopped tomatoes and
scampi. Simmer for a few minutes.

Cod Creole (see pages 113, 162)

SERVES 4
Calories per portion: 200
Preparation and cooking time: 55 minutes
Fat ★ Fibre ★ Protein ★★★ Iron ★★ Calcium ★ Vitamin C ★★★

Tomato Sauce for 4 (see recipe page 251)
1¼ lb (565 g) cod fillet, cut into four, or 4 × 5 oz (140 g) steaks
2 teaspoons brown sugar
Little tabasco, or ½ teaspoon chilli seasoning
2 teaspoons Worcestershire sauce
1 small green pepper, chopped

Make the tomato sauce and keep hot. Place the cod in a shallow ovenproof dish. Mix the sugar, Tabasco and Worcestershire sauce into the tomato sauce and pour over the cod. Sprinkle on the chopped pepper. Cover and cook at 180°C, Gas Mark 4, for 30 minutes, or until fish and peppers are cooked.

Monkfish Kebabs (see pages 119,130)

SERVES 4
Calories per portion: 300
Preparation and cooking time: 30 minutes
Fat ★★ Fibre ★ Protein ★★★ Iron ★★ Calcium ★ Vitamin C ★★★

½ quantity of Tomato Sauce (see recipe page 251)
1 dessertspoon clear honey
1 dessertspoon soy sauce
1 teaspoon mustard
1 lb (450 g) monkfish fillet, skinned and cubed
4 rashers lean bacon, cut into squares
1 small red pepper, cut into squares
1 small green pepper, cut into squares
12 button mushrooms
2 teaspoons corn oil

Make the tomato sauce (you could make a whole quantity and freeze the remaining half) and add to it the honey, soy sauce and mustard. Thread the fish, bacon and vegetables on to four long kebab sticks and brush with oil. Grill under a medium heat (or barbecue) for 10 to 12 minutes and serve with the hot sauce. (Monkfish is the best white fish for kebabs as it is meaty and doesn't flake, but you could use cod; it's almost as good.)

· POULTRY ·

Chicken Supreme (see page 108)

SERVES 4
Calories per portion: 250
Preparation and cooking time: 40 minutes
Fat ★ Fibre ★ Protein ★★★ Iron ★ Calcium ★★ Vitamin C ★

4 breasts chicken, boned and skinned
Salt and pepper
2 tablespoons dry/medium dry sherry, or lemon juice
⅓ pint (200 ml) chicken stock from cube
12 oz (340 g) button mushrooms, sliced
1 oz (30 g) low-fat spread
1 tablespoon flour
⅓ pint (200 ml) skimmed milk
2 fl oz (60 ml) Single cream substitute
4 sprigs parsley to garnish

Rub the chicken joints with salt and pepper and put in shallow baking-dish. Add the sherry, stock and mushrooms and bring to boil. Simmer gently for 25 minutes; remove chicken from stock and keep warm. Melt the spread in a saucepan and add the flour, cook for a minute or two. Mix the stock with the milk and gradually add to the saucepan to make a sauce, stirring all the time. Stir in the cream.

Check seasoning, and pour over chicken. Garnish with parsley. (Lemon juice instead of sherry will give an equally nice dish with a little more vitamin C.)

Chicken Tikka (see pages 108, 154, 162)

SERVES 4
Calories per portion: 200
Preparation and cooking time: 20 minutes (excluding marinating)
Fat ★ Fibre ★ Protein ★★★ Iron ★ Calcium ★★★ Vitamin C ★

¼ pint (150 ml) Greek strained yogurt
1 tablespoon lemon juice
2 tablespoons tikka paste
1 lb (450 g) skinless chicken meat, cubed

Mix the yogurt (if you can't get Greek, set low-fat yogurt will do) with the lemon juice and tikka paste in a bowl and add the chicken cubes. Leave for as long as possible, up to two hours, to marinate. (But even without, the dish still works.) Thread the coated chicken on kebab sticks and grill under a medium heat for 15 minutes − if there's any tikka left in the bowl, you can baste the chicken with it while it is cooking (spoon it over) and lengthen cooking time slightly. When the kebabs are slightly browned and the tikka is nearly dry, serve.

Chicken Tetrazzini (see pages 152, 153, 164)

SERVES 4
Calories per portion: 300
Preparation and cooking time: 40 minutes
Fat ★★ Fibre ★ Protein ★★★ Iron ★★ Calcium ★★★ Vitamin C ★

8 oz (225 g) cooked chicken meat, skinned and sliced
1 × 15 oz (425 g) can macaroni cheese
1 × 10 oz (285 g) can cream of chicken soup
8 oz (225 g) mushrooms, sliced
2 oz (55 g) Cheddar cheese, grated

Mix everything except the cheese together and pour into 3-pint (1·7 l) ovenproof dish. Cover and bake at 180°C, Gas Mark 4, for 35 minutes. Sprinkle cheese on top, and brown under grill.

Chicken Curry (see pages 119, 131, 163, 168)

SERVES 4
Calories per portion: 250
Preparation and cooking time: 35 minutes
Fat ★ Fibre ★ Protein ★★★ Iron ★★ Calcium ★ Vitamin C ★★

1 tablespoon corn oil
1 large onion, chopped
1 tablespoon curry powder of choice (more or less to taste)
1 lb (450 g) leftover cooked chicken meat
½ oz (15 g) seasoned flour
½ in garlic purée (optional)
2 oz (55 g) sultanas
½ pint (300 ml) chicken stock from cube
1 tablespoon tomato purée
1 dessert apple
½ a small tub natural set low-fat yogurt

Heat the oil in a frying pan and cook the onion until soft and just turning golden. Add the curry powder and cook, stirring, for a minute or two. Add the chicken, tossed in the flour; stir and cook for two more minutes. Add the garlic and sultanas, then the stock mixed with the tomato purée. Finally add the apple, sliced, and simmer for 25 minutes. Stir in the yogurt before serving.

Turkey Kebabs (see page 162)

SERVES 4
Calories per portion: 200
Preparation and cooking time: 25 minutes (excluding marinating)
Fat ★ Fibre ★ Protein ★★★ Iron ★★ Calcium ★ Vitamin C ★★★

1 quantity Barbecue Sauce (see recipe page 252)
12 oz (240 g) turkey meat
4 chipolatas
1 small onion, quartered and split
1 medium courgette, sliced
1 medium red pepper, cut into squares

Make the barbecue sauce and keep warm. Cut the turkey and chipolatas into bite-sized pieces and thread alternately on to metal skewers with the onion, courgette and pepper slices. If you have time, marinate the kebabs in the sauce for up to two hours, but if not it doesn't matter. Grill or barbecue the kebabs over a medium heat, basting with a little of the sauce from time to time. Serve with the rest of the sauce when the meat is thoroughly cooked through and browned.

Paradise Chicken (see page 150)

SERVES 4
Calories per portion: 300
Preparation and cooking time: 10 minutes
Fat ★★ Fibre ★ Protein ★★★ Iron ★ Calcium ★ Vitamin C ★

1 lb (450 g) cooked chicken or turkey meat, chopped
1 small glass white wine, or 2 tablespoons lemon juice
6 good tablespoons reduced-calorie mayonnaise
1 tablespoon corn or olive oil
1 tablespoon mild curry powder
1 tablespoon apricot jam (no lumps)
1 small carton natural yogurt
1 teaspoon onion powder
4 oz (115 g) chopped celery or dessert apple (optional)
½ oz (15 g) sultanas

Blend all ingredients together well and chill before serving.

· PASTA AND RICE ·

Macaroni Cheese (see pages 106, 154)

SERVES 4
Calories per portion: 350
Preparation and cooking time: 30 minutes
Fat ★ Fibre ★★ Protein ★★★ Iron ★ Calcium ★★★ Vitamin C ★

6 oz (175 g) raw weight macaroni
1 quantity Cheese Sauce (see recipe page 251)
Little nutmeg, grated
2 tomatoes
2 oz (55 g) reduced-fat Cheddar-style cheese

Cook the macaroni in a large pan of boiling, lightly salted water for 10 minutes or until just tender. Meanwhile, make the cheese sauce. Pour the drained macaroni and the sauce into an ovenproof dish with the nutmeg. Slice the tomatoes and arrange them nicely over the top of the macaroni cheese. Top with the grated cheese and bake uncovered at 200°C, Gas Mark 6, for 20 minutes, or until top is golden.

Tagliatelle with Ham (see pages 121, 133, 168)

SERVES 2

Calories per portion: 450

Preparation and cooking time: 15 minutes

Fat ★ Fibre ★★★ Protein ★★★ Iron ★★ Calcium ★★

Vitamin C ★★

4 oz (115 g) dry weight tagliatelle (half white, half green is best)

4 oz (115 g) frozen peas

4 oz (115 g) button mushrooms, sliced

4 fl oz (120 ml) chicken stock from cube

4 oz (115 g) boiled ham, chopped, or 1 × 4 oz (115 g) cooked lean gammon steak

Pinch of mixed herbs

Pepper and a little salt if necessary

4 fl oz (120 ml) Greek strained yogurt

1 tablespoon Parmesan cheese

Cook the tagliatelle in a large pan of boiling water for 10 minutes, or until just tender. Meanwhile, cook the peas and mushrooms in the stock in a frying-pan, then add the ham to heat through, plus the herbs and pepper. When you are ready to serve the drained pasta, add the yoghurt to the frying pan and warm through. Check seasoning and serve on the pasta with the cheese sprinkled over.

Pasta Shells with Tuna (see page 168)

SERVES 2
Calories per portion: 450
Preparation and cooking time: 15 minutes
Fat ★★ Fibre ★ Protein ★★★ Iron ★★★ Calcium ★★ Vitamin C ★

3 oz (85 g) dry weight pasta shells
½ small carton natural yogurt
4 tablespoons reduced-calorie mayonnaise
2 tablespoons lemon juice
1 tablespoon chopped parsley
Salt and pepper
1 × 7 oz (200 g) can tuna in brine, drained
2 size-3 eggs, hard-boiled

Cook the pasta shells in boiling water for 8 to 10 minutes,
until just tender, then drain and leave to cool. Mix together
the yogurt, mayonnaise, lemon juice, parsley and seasoning, and add the tuna, flaked, the eggs, chopped, and the
pasta. Toss and serve.
NOTE: A teaspoon of curry powder added to this dish
makes a nice change at no extra calories.

Spaghetti Bolognese (see pages 118, 168)

SERVES 4
Calories per portion: 450
Preparation and cooking time: 30 minutes
Fat ★★ Fibre ★★ Protein ★★★ Iron ★★★ Calcium ★★
Vitamin C ★★★

1 quantity Basic Mince (see recipe page 270)
1 small can chopped tomatoes
1 in garlic purée

8 oz (225 g) spaghetti
½ oz (15 g) low-fat spread
2 tablespoons Parmesan cheese

Cook the basic mince and add the tomatoes and garlic purée. Leave to simmer. Towards the end of cooking time, boil the spaghetti in a large pan of lightly salted water until just tender. Drain and toss in the low-fat spread. Serve topped with the sauce and cheese.

Lasagne (see pages 129, 168)

SERVES 4
Calories per portion: 550
Preparation and cooking time: 1 hour
Fat ★★★ Fibre ★★ Protein ★★★ Iron ★★★ Calcium ★★★
Vitamin C ★★★

1 quantity Basic Mince (see recipe page 270)
1 small can chopped tomatoes
½ in garlic purée
1 quantity Cheese Sauce (see recipe page 251)
6 oz (170 g) 'no need to pre-cook' lasagne leaves
2 oz (55 g) reduced-fat Cheddar-style cheese, grated

Make the basic mince and add the tomatoes and garlic. Make the cheese sauce. Add approx. ¼ pint (150 ml) extra water to the mince or as instructions on lasagne packet. In a lasagne or ovenproof dish put half the mince, then a layer of pasta, then the rest of the mince, then the rest of the pasta, and finally pour the cheese sauce over. Sprinkle with the grated cheese and bake at 200°C, Gas Mark 6, for 30 minutes, or until top is golden and bubbling.

Risotto (see pages 111, 154)

SERVES 4
Calories per portion: 350
Preparation and cooking time: 1 hour
Fat ★ Fibre ★★★ Protein ★★★ Iron ★★ Calcium ★ Vitamin C ★★

½ oz (15 g) low-fat spread
8 oz (225 g) long-grain rice
8 oz (225 g) chicken meat cut into bite-sized pieces
8 oz (225 g) button mushrooms, sliced
1 medium onion, finely chopped
½ in garlic purée (optional)
1¾ pint (1 l) chicken stock from cubes
1 tablespoon lemon juice
1 teaspoon turmeric powder, or 1 sachet saffron
Salt and pepper to taste
4 oz (115 g) peas
4 oz (115 g) peeled prawns
Lemon wedges to garnish

Melt the low-fat spread in a large non-stick pan, add the rice and stir to coat. Stir-fry for a minute or two. Add all the rest of the ingredients except the prawns and peas, bring to boil and simmer for 35 minutes uncovered, stirring occasionally. Add the peas and prawns, and cook for a further 5 minutes. Serve garnished with lemon wedges.
NOTE: Should risotto get too dry, add a little more stock during cooking.

· RED MEAT DISHES ·

Basic Minced Beef (see pages 111, 122, 133, 162)

SERVES 4
Calories per portion: 220
Preparation and cooking time: 30 minutes
Fat ★★ Fibre ★★ Protein ★★★ Iron ★★★ Calcium ★
Vitamin C ★★

1 tablespoon corn oil
1 large onion, finely chopped
1 lb (450 g) very lean minced beef
1 stick celery, chopped
1 large carrot, finely chopped
1 tablespoon tomato purée
1 teaspoon mixed herbs
½ pint (300 ml) beef stock made with gravy powder or granules
1 teaspoon Worcestershire sauce
Salt and pepper to taste

Heat the oil in a non-stick frying-pan and cook the onion over a medium heat until soft and transparent. Add the minced beef and cook until brown, stirring to break up the meat. Add vegetables and stir; add rest of ingredients and simmer for 20 minutes, or until beef is tender. Carefully spoon off any fat you can see on the top and discard (though if the mince was very lean there shouldn't be much).

NOTE: You can freeze this dish in full, half or quarter quantities for future use.

Moussaka (see pages 125, 136, 168)

SERVES 4
Calories per portion: 450
Preparation and cooking time: 1 hour 15 minutes
Fat ★★★ Fibre ★★★ Protein ★★★ Iron ★★★ Calcium ★★★
Vitamin C ★★★

1 large or 2 small aubergines (about 1 lb, 450 g)
1 quantity Basic Mince (see recipe page 270)
1 × 15 oz (425 g) tin tomatoes, chopped
1 quantity Cheese Sauce (see recipe page 251)
2 oz (55 g) reduced-fat Cheddar-style cheese, grated

Slice the aubergine (don't peel it) and blanch in boiling
water for 5 minutes. Drain and pat dry. Meanwhile, make
the basic mince and add the tomatoes, and make the cheese
sauce. In an ovenproof dish, put the mince, followed by the
aubergine slices and topped with the sauce. Sprinkle over
the grated cheese and bake at 200°C, Gas Mark 6, for 45
minutes, or until top is golden and bubbling.

Chilli Con Carne (see pages 111, 122, 134, 164)

SERVES 4
Calories per portion: 300
Preparation and cooking time: 45 minutes
Fat ★★ Fibre ★★★ Protein ★★★ Iron ★★★ Calcium ★★
Vitamin C ★★★

1 quantity Basic Mince (see recipe page 270)
1 × 15 oz (425 g) can red kidney beans
1 green pepper, finely chopped
1 teaspoon chilli powder (or to taste)

Make up the basic mince, add the beans, pepper and chilli
powder and simmer for a further 20 minutes or longer.

Beef Enchiladas (see pages 125, 136, 168)

SERVES 4
Calories per portion: 450
Preparation and cooking time: 30 minutes
Fat ★★★ Fibre ★★★ Protein ★★★ Iron ★★★ Calcium ★★
Vitamin C ★★★

1 × 12 oz (340 g) can corned beef
1 × 7½ oz (213 g) can red kidney beans, well drained
1 quantity Tomato Sauce (see recipe page 251)
Pinch chilli powder
12 Mexican tortillas, ready-made
1 tablespoon Parmesan cheese

Mash the corned beef and kidney beans in a bowl, together with a third of the tomato sauce, with the chilli. Fill the tortillas with a good spoonful of the mixture, roll up, and place in a shallow ovenproof dish. Pour the rest of the tomato sauce over the tortillas and bake at 180°C, Gas Mark 4, for 20 minutes, or until well heated through. Sprinkle over the cheese and serve.

Cottage Pie (see pages 105, 165)

SERVES 4
Calories per portion: 300
Preparation and cooking time: 1 hour
Fat ★★ Fibre ★★★ Protein ★★★ Iron ★★★ Calcium ★★
Vitamin C ★★★

1 quantity Basic Mince (see recipe page 270)
1 large carrot, finely chopped
1 lb (450 g) made-up weight instant mashed potato

Make up the basic mince, adding the extra carrot. Pour into

a 2½ pint (1·4 l) pie dish and top with the mashed potato. Bake at 200°C, Gas Mark 6, for 30 minutes, or until potato is crisp and golden.

Beef Goulash (see pages 112, 165)

SERVES 4

Calories per portion: 300
Preparation and cooking time: 2 hours
Fat ★★ Fibre ★★ Protein ★★★ Iron ★★★ Calcium ★★
Vitamin C ★★★

1 oz (30 g) flour
1 tablespoon paprika
1 lb (450 g) lean, trimmed stewing steak, cubed
1 tablespoon corn oil
1 large green pepper, sliced
1 large onion, sliced
4 oz (115 g) mushrooms
1 × 15 oz (425 g) can tomatoes
¼ pint (150 ml) beef stock from cube
Salt and pepper to taste
4 oz (115 g) thick strained yogurt

Mix together the flour and paprika and coat the beef. Heat the oil in a large pan and brown the cubes of beef a few at a time. Remove and keep warm. Now stir round the pepper and onion, then add all remaining ingredients except yogurt. Bring to boil, cover and simmer for 1 hour 45 minutes, or until beef is tender. Stir in yogurt before serving.

Beef Stroganoff (see pages 112, 165)

SERVES 4
Calories per portion: 300
Preparation and cooking time: 20 minutes
Fat ★★ Fibre ★ Protein ★★★ Iron ★★★ Calcium ★
Vitamin C ★★★

½ oz (15 g) butter
1 onion, finely chopped
8 oz (225 g) button mushrooms, sliced
1¼ lb (565 g) beef fillet or rump, very thinly sliced into
bite-sized pieces
½ oz (15 g) flour
Pinch cayenne pepper
2 tablespoons dry sherry
⅓ pint (200 ml) beef stock from cube
1 × 5 oz (140 g) carton soured cream
Little salt if necessary

Melt the butter in a non-stick frying pan and fry the onion
until soft and just turning golden. Add the mushrooms and
stir-fry over a fairly high heat for a minute or two. Add the
beef, tossed in the flour seasoned with cayenne, and stir-fry
for 3 to 4 minutes. Add the sherry and cook for 1 minute.
Add the stock, bubble for 1 minute, and finally add the
soured cream. Warm through and serve.

Beef Stir-Fry (see pages 106, 162)

SERVES 4
Calories per portion: 200
Preparation and cooking time: 20 minutes
Fat ★ Fibre ★ Protein ★★★ Iron ★★★ Calcium ★ Vitamin C ★★★

1 tablespoon corn oil
12 oz (340 g) rump steak, cut into thin strips
4 oz (115 g) mushrooms, sliced
4 oz (115 g) sweetcorn
8 spring onions, chopped
1 red pepper, sliced
1 tablespoon sherry
2 teaspoons clear honey
Pinch ground ginger
1 tablespoon soy sauce
1 tablespoon cornflour mixed with 4 tablespoons water

In a large non-stick frying-pan or wok, heat the oil and stir-fry the beef for a minute or two over a high heat until well browned. Add the vegetables and stir-fry for another 2 minutes. Add the sherry and honey and stir. Finally, add the ginger, soy sauce and cornflour mixture, bring all to boil and thicken. Serve.

Beef Curry (see pages 166, 169)

SERVES 4
Calories per portion: 350
Preparation and cooking time: 2 hours
Fat ★★★ Fibre ★ Protein ★★★ Iron ★★★ Calcium ★
Vitamin C ★★★

½ oz (15 g) butter
1 dessertspoon corn oil

1 large onion, chopped
1¼ lb (565 g) extra-lean braising steak, cubed
½ in garlic purée (optional)
1 level tablespoon (more or less to taste) Madras curry powder
1 small can tomatoes, chopped
1 heaped tablespoon flour
4 oz (115 g) potato
6 oz (170 g) broccoli or cauliflower, broken into small florets
1 level dessertspoon tomato purée
1 oz (30 g) raisins
1 teaspoon sugar
¾ pint (450 ml) good strong beef stock (skimmed of fat if home-made)
Salt and pepper to taste

Melt the butter and oil together in a flameproof casserole or large non-stick pan, add onion and soften. Add beef and brown lightly. Add garlic (if using) and curry powder and stir for a minute. Add flour, stir again, and let cook for a few minutes. Add rest of ingredients and simmer on hob or in a slow oven for 1 hour 45 minutes.

NOTE: You can use leftover lean beef in this recipe. There is no need to brown it: instead, add with the stock and reduce cooking time by 45 minutes.

Lamb Kebabs (see pages 106, 163)

SERVES 4

Calories per portion: 250

Preparation and cooking time: 30 minutes

Fat ★★ Fibre ★ Protein ★★★ Iron ★★ Calcium ★
Vitamin C ★★★

12 oz (340 g) lean fillet of lamb, cubed
4 × 1 oz (30 g) back bacon rashers, trimmed of fat
1 medium onion, quartered and split
1 × 4 oz (115 g) courgette, sliced
1 green pepper, cut into squares
2 tomatoes, quartered
1 quantity Barbecue Sauce (see recipe page 252)

Divide the meat and vegetables between four long kebab sticks and grill or barbecue for 15 minutes. Serve with the heated sauce poured over.

NOTE: You could also use pork fillet instead of the lamb in this dish.

Sweet and Sour Pork (see pages 123, 134, 166, 169)

SERVES 4

Calories per portion: 350

Preparation and cooking time: 1 hour 15 minutes

Fat ★★ Fibre ★ Protein ★★★ Iron ★★ Calcium ★ Vitamin C ★

1 tablespoon corn oil
1¼ lb (565 g) lean fillet of pork, cubed
¾ pint (450 ml) chicken stock from cube
Salt and pepper to taste
1 red pepper, sliced
1 green pepper, sliced

1 × 8 oz (225 g) can pineapple chunks in natural juice
or water
1 tablespoon soy sauce
2 level tablespoons soft brown sugar
2 level tablespoons vinegar
1 level tablespoon cornflour

Heat the oil in a flameproof casserole and brown the pork.
Add the stock and seasoning and simmer at 180°C, Gas
Mark 4, for 1 hour. Return casserole dish to hob, add
peppers and pineapple and simmer for a few minutes. Mix
together the soya sauce, sugar, vinegar and cornflour, then
add to casserole. Stir until sauce thickens and bubbles.
Serve.

Liver Paprika (see pages 166, 169)

SERVES 4
Calories per portion: 350
Preparation and cooking time: 20 minutes
Fat ★★★ Fibre ★ Protein ★★★ Iron ★★★ Calcium ★
Vitamin C ★★★

½ oz (15 g) butter
1 tablespoon corn oil
1 lb (450 g) lamb's liver, cut into very thin, bite-sized
pieces
1 large onion, very finely chopped
1 green pepper, sliced
Salt and pepper
1 good tablespoon paprika, preferably Hungarian
1 × 4¼ fl oz (130 ml) carton soured cream

5 fl oz (1 glass, 150 ml) red wine, or equivalent cooking wine

Even if you think you hate liver, you will love this rich, creamy dish – as long as you don't overcook the liver and toughen it – so give it a try!

Melt the butter and oil in a frying-pan and over a high heat, very quickly brown the liver (for not more than a minute or two), then transfer using a slotted spatula on to a plate. Add the onion and pepper to the pan and, with heat lowered, cook for 5 to 10 minutes until onions are soft and transparent and peppers cooked through. Add the salt and pepper and paprika, stir and cook for a minute. Add the wine and let it bubble. Return liver to pan and stir round for a minute, then pour in the soured cream and let it warm as it mixes with the wine juices. Serve straight away.

Corned Beef Hash (see pages 116, 128)

SERVES 4

Calories per portion: 400

Preparation and cooking time: 15 minutes

Fat ★★★ Fibre ★★ Protein ★★★ Iron ★★★ Calcium ★

Vitamin C ★★

1 oz (30 g) butter
1 tablespoon corn oil
1 × 12 oz (340 g) can corned beef
1 lb (450 g) made-up weight instant mashed potato
1 small onion, finely chopped
1 size-3 egg, beaten
1 tablespoon skimmed milk

Melt the butter and oil in a non-stick frying-pan. Meanwhile, mash up together all the rest of the ingredients and make four patties. Fry the patties over a medium heat for 5 minutes a side, or until they are golden brown.

Quick Boston Baked Beans (see pages 104, 165)

SERVES 4
Calories per portion: 300
Preparation and cooking time: 30 minutes
Fat ★★ Fibre ★★★ Protein ★★ Iron ★★★ Calcium ★★
Vitamin C ★

8 skinless pork chipolatas, grilled, or 8 oz (255 g) lean ham, chopped
1 × 1¼ lb (565 g) can baked beans in tomato sauce
1 level tablespoon dark brown sugar
2 tablespoons Worcestershire sauce
2 teaspoons made mustard

Cut the chipolatas into bite-sized pieces. Pour the beans into a lightly oiled ovenproof dish and add the rest of the ingredients, stirring to mix well. Cover and bake at 180°C, Gas Mark 4, until the beans are simmering – about 20 minutes.

Toad in the Hole (see pages 116, 127, 169)

SERVES 4
Calories per portion: 400
Preparation and cooking time: 45 minutes
Fat ★★ Fibre ★ Protein ★★ Iron ★★ Calcium ★★ Vitamin C ★

1 tablespoon corn oil
8 large low-fat pork sausages
2 size-3 eggs
½ pint (300 ml) skimmed milk
Little salt and pepper
4 oz (115 g) plain flour

Brush a baking-tin with the corn oil and add the sausages. Cook at 220°C, Gas Mark 7, for 5 to 10 minutes. Meanwhile, make a batter by beating the eggs, milk and salt into the flour. Pour this over the sausages and return to oven for 30 to 40 minutes, or until well risen and golden.

APPENDIX
THE JUNK FOOD DIRECTORY

Food	Calories	Protein (g)	Fat (g)	Fibre (g)	Calcium (mg)	Iron (mg)	Vitamin C (mg)	Added sugar (g)
Alcoholic drinks:								
Beer, ½ pint (300 ml)	90	1	—	—	30	tr	—	6
Lager, ½ pint (300 ml)	90	1	—	—	30	tr	—	6
All spirits, 1 measure	50	tr	—	—	tr	tr	—	tr
Stout, ½ pint (300 ml)	100	tr	tr	—	20	tr	—	11
Wine, white, 5 fl oz (150 ml)	100	tr	—	—	13	0·75	—	1
Wine, sweet, 5 fl oz (150 ml)	140	tr	—	—	21	0·8	—	9
Wine, red, 5 fl oz (150 ml)	100	tr	—	—	10	1·3	—	0·5
Almonds, shelled, 1 oz (30 g)	158	5	4	4	75	1	—	—
Apple, 1 average	40	tr	tr	2·5	6	0·5	7	—
Apple juice, 4 fl oz (120 ml)	40	tr	—	tr	6	tr	0–5	—
Apple pie, 1 average 5 oz (140 g) portion	350	6	15	2	50	1·5	5	15
Apple sauce, 1 tablespoon	20	tr	tr	tr	2	tr	tr	4
Apricot, 1 fresh	20	tr	tr	1·5	10	0·25	5	—
Apricots, dried, 1 oz (30 g)	50	1·3	tr	6	25	1	—	—

Artichoke, Jerusalem, boiled, average 4 oz (115 g) portion	18	1.6	tr	tr	30	0.4	2	–
Asparagus, 1 spear	5	1	tr	0.4	6	0.25	5	–
Aubergine, 1 average, 8 oz (225 g)	30	1.5	tr	5	20	0.75	10	–
Avocado, ½ a medium	200	3.5	4.5	2	15	1.25	15	–
Bacon, 1 back rasher, well grilled or fried	80	9	3.5	–	2	0.25	–	–
Bacon, 1 streaky rasher, well grilled or fried	50	7	2.75	–	1	0.2	–	–
Bacon steak, grilled, 4 oz (115 g)	120	20	2.25	–	7	1	–	–
Bagel, 1 average	150	2	tr	1	40	0.7	–	tr
Baked beans, 5 oz (140 g) portion	110	7	tr	10	67	2	–	7
Banana, 1 average	80	1	tr	4	7	0.5	10	–
Beansprouts, 1 oz (30 g)	8	1	–	1	5	0.5	1	–
Beef, lean minced, raw 1 oz (30 g)	45	5	4	–	4	1	–	–
Beef, lean roast, 1 average slice (1 oz, 30 g)	45	10	4	–	2	0.5	–	–
Beef, mince, stewed with onion and gravy, 1 average portion, 8 oz (225 g)	220	21	15	1	40	4	5	tr
Beefburger, 2 oz (55 g) in bap, average	250	16	6.25	1.25	60	2.2	–	tr
Beefburger, quarterpounder (no bun), well grilled or fried	240	24	10	–	30	3	–	–
Beefburger, quarterpounder in bap, average	370	28	11	1	75	3.7	–	tr

Food	Calories	Protein (g)	Fat (g)	Fibre (g)	Calcium (mg)	Iron (mg)	Vitamin C (mg)	Added sugar (g)
Beefsteak and kidney pie, 1 individual (5 oz, 142 g)	400	13	30	tr	75	3·5	–	tr
Beetroot, cooked, 1 oz (30 g) – 1 small root	12	tr	tr	0·25	10	tr	1·5	–
Biscuits:								
Choc chip cookie, 1	50	0·5	1	tr	3	0·2	–	2·5
Digestive, 1 large	75	1·5	3	0·75	14	0·5	–	2·5
Digestive, chocolate coated, 1 large	95	1	4	0·75	16	0·25	–	4
Gingernut, 1	45	0·5	1·5	0·2	13	0·4	–	3·5
Rich Tea, 1	35	0·5	1·5	0·2	10	0·15	–	1·8
Shortcake, 1	95	1	4	0·3	15	0·25	–	2·5
Black Forest Gateau, 1 average slice, 4 oz (115 g)	225	4	15	0·5	50	1	–	15
Blackberries, 1 oz (30 g)	8	0·4	tr	2	18	0·25	5	–
Blackcurrants, 1 oz (30 g) raw	8	tr	tr	2	16	0·35	56	–
Blackcurrant cordial, ½ pint (300 ml)	80	tr	tr	–	3	tr	60	18
Black pudding, fried, 1 oz (30 g)	85	3·5	6	–	10	5·5	–	–
Branflakes, 1 oz (30 g)	92	2·5	0·5	4	tr	11	–	4·5
Brazil nuts, 1 oz (30 g)	180	4	19	1	50	0·8	–	–
Bread:								
Bap, 1	130	4·2	1·25	1·25	45	0·7	–	tr
Brown, 1 oz (30 g)	65	2·25	0·5	1·5	28	0·6	–	–

French, 1 oz (30 g)	85	2.5	0.5	1	29	0.5	—	—
Granary, 1 oz (30 g)	70	2.5	1	2	28	0.6	—	—
Malt, 1 oz (30 g)	70	2.25	0.75	1.5	28	1	—	2
Pitta, 1 whole	180	3	tr	3	75	1.25	—	—
Rye, 1 oz (30 g)	90	3	tr	1.5	25	0.5	—	—
White, soft grain, 1 slice from medium loaf	80	2.5	0.5	1.1	46	0.75	tr	tr
White, 1 oz (30 g)	70	2.25	0.5	1	29	0.5	—	tr
Wholemeal, 1 oz (30 g)	60	2.25	0.5	2.5	15	0.75	—	—
Bun, 1 currant	150	3.5	3.5	tr	45	1.25	60	7
Broccoli, 4 oz (115 g) serving	20	3	tr	4	80	1	40	—
Brussels sprouts, 4 oz (115 g) serving	18	3	tr	3	25	0.5	—	—
Butter, 1 oz (30 g)	210	—	23	—	4	tr	20	—
Cabbage, 4 oz (115 g) serving	16	2	tr	3	38	0.5	—	—
Cake, 2 oz (55 g) slice:								
Fancy chocolate	250	3	15	1	65	0.75	—	10
Jam sponge	140	2	7	0.5	20	0.5	—	11
Rich fruit	165	3	10	2	40	1.5	—	7
Carrots, 4 oz (115 g) serving	20	1	3	50	0.75	10	25	—
Cashew nuts, 1 oz (30 g)	160	5	14	2	12	1	3	—
Cauliflower, 4 oz (115 g) serving	12	2	tr	2	20	0.5	—	—
Celery, 1 stick	5	tr	tr	0.75	20	0.25	—	—
Cheese:								
Brie, 1 oz (30 g)	88	5	7	—	106	tr	—	—
Camembert, 1 oz (30 g)	88	5	7	—	106	tr	—	—

Food	Calories	Protein (g)	Fat (g)	Fibre (g)	Calcium (mg)	Iron (mg)	Vitamin C (mg)	Added sugar (g)
Cheddar, 1 oz (30 g)	120	7	9	—	224	tr	—	—
Cheddar-style, low-fat, 1 oz (30 g)	70	8	4	—	230	tr	—	—
Cheese spread, 1 triangle, ½ oz (15 g)	40	3	3.5	—	75	tr	—	—
Cheshire, 1 oz (30 g)	110	7	8	—	224	tr	—	—
Cottage, 1 small carton	105	14	4	—	70	tr	—	—
Danish Blue, 1 oz (30 g)	100	5	8	—	88	tr	—	—
Edam, 1 oz (25 g)	90	7	7	—	220	tr	—	—
Gorgonzola, 1 oz (30 g)	110	5	7	—	88	tr	—	—
Skimmed-milk soft, 1 small carton	100	15	4	—	70	tr	—	—
Cherries, 1 oz (30 g)	12	tr	tr	0.5	5	tr	5	—
Chicken, 1 average joint, baked or grilled	160	24	6	—	8	0.8	—	—
Chicken, lean roast, 1 oz (30 g) slice	40	6	1.5	—	2	0.2	—	—
Chicken roll, 1 slice	38	5	1.75	—	2	0.2	—	—
Chips, 4 oz (115 g):								
Average cut	280	4	20	1	15	1	10	—
Crinkle cut	320	4	24	1	15	1	8	—
Extra thick	180	4	9	1	15	1	12	—
French fries	330	4	25	1	15	1	8	—
Oven chips	200	4	10	1	15	1	10	—
Chocolate, milk, 1 oz (30 g)	150	2	7	—	50	0.4	—	12

Chocolate, plain, 1 oz (30 g)	150	1	7	–	10	0·6	–	12
Chocolate bars:								
Dairy Milk, 1½ oz (40 g)	210	3	10	–	75	0·6	–	18
Kit Kat, 4 fingers	245	n/k	n/k	tr	n/k	1	–	n/k
Mars, standard	295	3·8	11·5	tr	110	1	1·2	42
Wispa, standard	200	n/k	n/k	–	n/k	0·5	–	n/k
Yorkie, 2⅓ oz (67 g)	360	5	16	–	120	1	–	28
Coca Cola, 1 can	130	–	–	–	13	–	–	34
Cocoa powder, 1 dessertspoon	30	2	3	tr	14	1	–	–
Coconut, 1 oz (30 g)	100	1	10	1	3	0·6	tr	–
Cod, cooked without fat, 1 oz (30 g)	22	5	tr	–	6	tr	–	–
Cod in batter, average portion, 7 oz (200 g)	470	44	20	1	162	1	–	–
Coffee, 1 cup, black	2	tr	tr	–	tr	tr	–	2
Coleslaw, ready made, 1 small tub	150	3	13·5	3	60	0·6	25	–
Coley, cooked without fat, 1 oz (25 g)	21	5	tr	–	6	tr	–	–
Corn on the cob, 1	100	4·5	2·5	5	5	1	10	–
Corned beef, 1 oz (30 g) slice	60	7·5	3·5	–	4	0·8	–	2
Cornflakes, 1 oz (30 g)	100	2·5	tr	0·5	5	2	–	–
Cornflour, 1 heaped teaspoon	15	tr	tr	–	tr	tr	–	–
Courgette, 1 average, raw, 3 oz, (85 g)	10	1	tr	1·5	25	0·5	10	–
Crab, fresh, 1 small (edible contents)	115	20	5	–	25	1	–	–
Crabmeat, canned, 1 oz (30 g)	22	5	tr	–	33	0·75	–	–

Food	Calories	Protein (g)	Fat (g)	Fibre (g)	Calcium (mg)	Iron (mg)	Vitamin C (mg)	Added sugar (g)
Cream, 1 oz (30 g):								
Clotted	165	0.75	18	—	n/k	n/k	—	—
Double	125	0.4	13	—	14	tr	tr	—
Single	60	0.67	6	—	13	tr	0.4	—
Soured	50	0.75	5	—	22	n/k	—	n/k
Cream, non-dairy, 1 oz (30 g)	55	—	7	1.5	n/k	n/k	—	0.3
Crispbread, rye, 1	30	1	0.2	0.5	n/k	0.37	—	0.75
Crispbread, wheat, 1	30	4	0.75	3.5	5	0.54	—	tr
Crisps, low fat, 1 pack	105	2	6.5	3.5	6	0.63	5	tr
Crisps, ready salted, 1 pack	135	2	10	tr	11	0.63	5	tr
Cucumber, 1 oz (30 g)	3	tr	tr	—	11	tr	2	—
Custard, ready to serve, ½ can (4 oz, 115 g)	110	4	4	—	6	tr	—	10
Dates, dried, 1	10	tr	tr	1	140	0.2	—	—
Doughnut, jam, 1	225	4	10	1	7	1.25	—	10
Duck, well cooked, flesh only, 1 oz (30 g)	52	7	3	—	50	0.75	—	—
Egg, 1 × size 3, fried in a little corn oil in non-stick pan and well drained	100	6.5	7.75	—	1	1	—	—
Egg, raw, boiled or poached, 1 × size 3	80	6.5	5.5	—	28	1	—	—
Egg, Scotch, 1 average (4 oz, 113 g)	280	12	20	—	56	1.7	—	—

Figs, 1	20	0.5	tr	1.5	18	0.25	–	–
Fish cake, dry-fried or grilled, 1	80	4	4	–	35	0.5	–	–
Fish fingers, dry-fried or grilled, 2	100	6	5	–	20	0.3	–	–
Fish in butter sauce, 1 individual packet	155	18	5.5	–	n/k	n/k	–	–
Fish paste, 1 × 1 oz (35 g) pot	65	6	3.5	–	100	3	–	–
Flour, 1 tablespoon	50	1.5	0.2	0.5	22	0.36	–	–
Frankfurter, 1 (1 oz, 30 g)	60	2	5	–	7	0.33	–	–
French dressing, 1 tablespoon	100	–	11	–	tr	–	–	1
Gammon, boiled, lean, 1 oz (30 g) slice	46	8	1.5	–	2.8	0.5	–	–
Gammon steak, fat trimmed, well grilled, 6 oz (170 g)	300	50	9	–	17	2.5	–	n/k
Ginger beer, 11¼ fl oz (330 ml) can	160	–	–	–	–	tr	–	13
Grapefruit, canned, including syrup, 4 oz (115 g)	60	0.5	tr	0.4	17	0.7	10	–
Grapefruit, canned and drained, 4 oz (115 g)	20	tr	tr	0.5	8	0.15	20	–
Grapefruit, half fresh	15	tr	tr	0.5	7	0.12	30	–
Grapes, 1 oz (30 g)	17	tr	tr	0.25	5	tr	1	–
Gravy, thick, 1 tablespoon	20	0.5	2	–	tr	tr	–	–
Gravy from cube, 1 tablespoon	2	tr	tr	–	tr	tr	–	–
Haddock, average portion, deep-fried in batter, (8 oz, 225 g)	320	40	15	tr	200	2.2	–	–
Haddock, cooked without fat, 4 oz (115 g)	73	17	0.6	–	18	0.6	–	–

Food	Calories	Protein (g)	Fat (g)	Fibre (g)	Calcium (mg)	Iron (mg)	Vitamin C (mg)	Added sugar (g)
Ham, extra lean, 1 oz (30 g)	25	4	0.5	–	n/k	n/k	–	–
Ham, lean, boiled, 1 oz (30 g) slice	40	5	2	–	2	0.3	–	–
Hazelnuts, shelled, 1 oz (30 g)	105	2	10	1.7	12	1.3	tr	–
Herring, cooked without fat, 8 oz (225 g)	470	33	37	–	66	1.6	–	–
Honey, 1 tablespoon	60	–	tr	–	tr	tr	–	15
Hot dog, 1 average	160	5.2	5.7	1.1	49	1	–	1
Ice cream, choc ice, 1	125	3	5	–	100	tr	–	15
Ice cream, Cornetto, 1 strawberry	200	2.5	8	–	n/k	tr	–	n/k
Ice cream, vanilla, 1 scoop (2 oz, 55 g)	90	2	3.5	–	75	tr	tr	12
Ice cream, vanilla, 1 soft cone	80	1.5	3.5	–	70	–	–	12
Ice cream cone, cone only	10	tr	tr	–	tr	–	–	1.5
Ice lolly, average	60	tr	–	–	–	–	–	14
Icing, royal, 1 oz (30 g)	85	tr	–	–	–	–	–	21
Instant whip, made up, ¼ packet	150	5	7.5	–	140	0.16	–	–
Jam, for 1 slice bread ½ oz (10 g)	30	–	–	tr	2	tr	1	7
Jam tart, 1 average	130	1.2	5.2	0.6	21	0.5	1	13
Jelly, average serving 5 oz (140 g)	90	2.1	–	–	10	0.6	–	21
Kidney, lamb's, 1 whole	50	9	1.5	–	5.6	4	–	–
Kipper, well grilled, 1 average	250	30	13	–	76	1.6	–	–
Kiwifruit, 1	30	0.7	tr	1.5	15	tr	60	–

Lamb:

Lamb chop, trimmed and well grilled, 1 average	190	25	12	—	9	2·1	—	—
Lamb, fillet, lean, raw, 1 oz (30 g)	40	6	2·4	—	2	0·5	—	—
Lean roast leg, 1 average slice (1 oz, 30 g)	50	8	2	—	2·2	0·75	—	—
Roast shoulder, 1 slice, 1 oz (30 g)	88	5·6	7·3	—	2 5	0·5	—	—
Lard, 1 oz (30 g)	250	tr	27·72	—	tr	—	—	—
Leeks, 4 oz (115 g) serving	36	2	tr	6	60	2	20	8
Lemon, 1 whole, excluding peel	15	0·5	tr	2	60	tr	80	18
Lemon curd, 1 oz	80	tr	tr	—	tr	tr	tr	tr
Lemonade, 11½ fl oz (330 ml) can	90	—	—	—	—	—	—	—
Lentils, raw 1 oz (30 g) or cooked 3 oz (85 g)	85	6·6	tr	3·25	11	2·1	—	—
Lettuce, average serving, 2 oz (55 g)	4	0·4	tr	0·5	8	0·35	6	—
Liver, dry-fried or grilled, 4 oz	200	20	10	—	7	9·5	10	—
Liver sausage, 1 oz (30 g)	85	3·6	7·5	—	7	1·8	—	—
Low-fat spread (e.g. Gold), 1 oz (30 g)	105	1·8	11	—	—	—	—	—
Luncheon meat, 1 oz (30 g)	85	3·5	7·5	—	4	0·3	—	—
Mackerel, baked, 1 small fish (8 oz, 225 g)	320	45	23	—	60	2·5	—	—
Malted drink made with whole milk, ⅓ pint (200 ml)	150	4	5·6	—	225	n/k	1	n/k
Mandarins, canned in juice, ½ × 10½ oz (300 g) tin	45	tr	tr	0·5	15	0·4	14	—
Mangetout, 4 oz (115 g) serving	45	6	tr	7	25	1·5	15	—
Mango, 1 whole	100	1	tr	2	15	0·75	45	—

Food	Calories	Protein (g)	Fat (g)	Fibre (g)	Calcium (mg)	Iron (mg)	Vitamin C (mg)	Added sugar (g)
Maple syrup, 1 tablespoon	50	tr	tr	–	n/k	n/k	–	14
Margarine, 1 oz (30 g)	205	–	22·8	–	1	tr	–	–
Marmalade, for 1 slice bread, ⅔ oz (10 g)	25	–	tr	tr	tr	tr	1	7
Marzipan, 1 oz (30 g)	125	21	6·2	1·6	30	0·5	–	12·5
Mayonnaise, 1 tablespoon	120	tr	12	–	tr	tr	–	–
Meringue, 1 case	65	1	–	–	tr	tr	–	14
Milk, 1 pint (600 ml):								
Semi-skimmed	265	19	4·5	–	700	0·3	8	26
Skimmed	195	19	tr	–	720	0·3	9	28
Whole	380	18	20	–	676	0·3	8	26
Milk, dried, 1 tablespoon, low-fat	50	5	tr	–	160	tr	tr	7
Milkshake, full fat, ½ pint (300 ml)	375	10	12	–	350	tr	tr	n/k
Milkshake, low-fat, (200 ml) carton	120	6	tr	–	230	tr	tr	n/k
Mince pie, 1 average	215	2	10	1·5	38	0·8	–	15
Mincemeat, 1 oz (30 g)	65	tr	1·2	1	8	0·5	tr	13
Mint sauce, 1 teaspoon	5	–	–	tr	tr	tr	–	1
Monkfish, cooked without fat, 1 oz (30 g)	20	5	tr	–	6	tr	–	–
Muesli, 1 oz (30 g)	105	3·6	2·1	2	56	1·3	tr	13
Muesli bar, 1 average, 1 oz (30 g)	115	2·2	4	1·2	n/k	n/k	–	13
Mushrooms, fried, 1 oz (30 g) cooked weight	60	0·5	6	0·75	tr	0·3	1	–

Mushrooms, raw, 1 oz (30 g)	4	0.5	tr	0.75	tr	0.3	1	—
Mussels, shelled, 1 oz (30 g)	25	4	tr	—	50	2	—	—
Nectarine, 1	50	1	tr	2.5	4	0.5	8	—
Noodles, boiled, 4 oz (115 g) serving	132	4.5	tr	1	10	0.5	—	—
Pot Noodles, 1 tub	300	n/k	n/k	1.5	n/k	n/k	tr	5
Nuts, chopped, mixed, 1 oz (30 g)	160	3	15	1.2	30	0.5	—	—
Oats, porridge, made up, 8 oz (225 g) serving	100	3.15	2	1.6	13.5	1.1	—	—
Oats, raw, 1 oz (30 g)	112	3.4	2.4	2	15	1.1	—	—
Oil, vegetable, all kinds, 1 oz (30 ml)	251	tr	27.97	—	tr	tr	—	—
Onion, raw, 1 small, 4 oz (115 g)	23	0.9	tr	1.3	31	0.3	10	—
Onion, sliced and fried, in oil, 1 oz (30 g) cooked weight	95	0.5	9.3	1.2	17	0.17	tr	—
Onion, spring, 1 medium	10	0.9	tr	0.85	39	0.3	7	—
Orange, 1	50	1.1	tr	2.8	57	0.4	70	—
Orange juice, 5 fl oz (¼ pint, 150 ml) serving	50	0.6	—	—	12	0.5	50	—
Oxtail stew, including bone, 1 × 11 oz (310 g) serving	275	35	15	—	15	4.2	—	—
Parsnips, boiled, 4 oz (115 g) serving	56	1.3	tr	2.5	36	0.5	10	—
Pasta, all types, boiled 1 oz (30 g) cooked weight	33	1.2	tr	tr	2	tr	—	—
Pastry, shortcrust, 1 oz (30 g) cooked weight	148	1.9	9	0.7	30	0.5	—	—

Food	Calories	Protein (g)	Fat (g)	Fibre (g)	Calcium (mg)	Iron (mg)	Vitamin C (mg)	Added sugar (g)
Pâté, liver, 1 oz (30 g)	80	4	5·4	–	6	2·2	–	–
Peach, 1	40	0·7	tr	1·5	5	0·5	9	–
Peach slices in juice, 4 oz (115 g) serving	40	0·7	tr	1·5	5	0·5	5	5
Peach slices in syrup, 4 oz (115 g) serving	90	0·4	tr	1	4	0·4	4	14
Peanuts, shelled, 1 oz (30 g)	160	7	13	2·35	17	0·5	–	–
Pear, 1 medium	50	tr	tr	3	10	0·2	3	–
Peas. 4 oz (115 g):								
Canned, drained	47	4·6	0·3	6·3	24	1·6	8	–
Frozen, boiled	41	5·4	0·4	12	31	1·4	13	–
Split (cooked weight)	118	8·3	0·3	5·1	11	1·7	–	–
Peppers, green, raw, 1 oz (30 g)	4	tr	tr	0·25	2·5	tr	28	–
Pheasant, roast, ½ an average bird	240	35	10	–	50	9	–	–
Pickle, sweet, 1 tablespoon	20	tr	tr	0·25	3	0·3	–	5
Pineapple, canned in syrup, 4 oz (115 g)	75	0·3	tr	0·9	13	0·4	12	9
Pineapple, fresh, 1 slice	20	0·25	tr	0·6	6	0·2	12	–
Pizza, cheese and tomato, 1 individual 3½ oz (100 g)	200	9	11	0·5	220	1	3	–
Pizza, French bread, 1	320	15	12	2·5	n/k	n/k	n/k	6·7
Plaice, breaded and fried, 1 average portion 6 oz (170 g)	380	30	23	–	112	1·3	–	–
Plaice, cooked without fat, 1 average fillet 5 oz, (140 g)	130	27	2·6	–	50	0·9	–	–
Plum, 1 dessert	15	tr	tr	0·7	4	0·14	1	–

Popcorn, 1 individual bag, savoury (no oil)	265	n/k	n/k	tr	n/k	n/k	–	–
Pork, roast, lean only, 1 oz (30 g) slice	50	8·5	2	–	2·5	0·36	–	–
Pork chop, trimmed and well grilled, 1 average	300	45	15	–	12·6	1·7	–	–
Pork crackling, average portion ½oz (15 g)	100	tr	12	–	tr	tr	–	–
Pork fillet, raw 1 oz (30 g)	40	5·8	2	–	2·2	0·25	–	–
Pork pie, 1 individual, 5 oz (145 g)	545	14	39	–	68	2	–	–
Potatoes, 4 oz (115 g) serving: Instant mashed with added vitamin C	70	2	tr	3·6	20	0·5	15	–
Mashed with milk and butter	120	1·5	5	0·9	12	0·3	8	–
New, boiled	76	1·6	tr	2	5	0·4	18	–
Old, boiled	80	1·4	tr	1	4	0·3	10	–
Potatoes, baked, 6 oz (170 g) potato	150	4	tr	3·7	13	1·2	15	–
Potatoes, roast, 1 average chunk	80	1·4	2·5	tr	5	0·3	5	–
Prawns, peeled, 1 oz (30 g)	30	6·3	0·5	–	42	0·3	tr	–
Prunes, 1 oz (30 g)	45	0·67	tr	4·5	10	0·8	tr	–
Quiche, average 5 oz (140 g) slice	400	14	28	tr	260	1·3	–	–
Radish, 1	1	tr	tr	tr	3	0·13	2	–
Raisins, 1 oz, (30 g)	68	tr	tr	2	17	0·5	–	–
Raspberries, 4 oz (115 g) serving	28	0·9	tr	7·4	41	1·2	25	–

Food	Calories	Protein (g)	Fat (g)	Fibre (g)	Calcium (mg)	Iron (mg)	Vitamin C (mg)	Added sugar (g)
Rhubarb, stewed, 4 oz (115 g) incl. sugar	45	0.5	tr	2.2	84	0.3	7	10
Rice, 4 oz (115 g) serving:								
Brown, boiled	118	2.2	0.9	3	3	0.5	–	–
White, boiled	120	2.2	0.3	0.8	1	0.2	–	–
White, fried	230	2.2	12	0.8	1	0.2	–	–
Rice Krispies, 1 oz (30 g)	104	1.6	0.56	1.26	2	0.19	–	2.5
Rice pudding, canned, $\frac{1}{4}$ × 16 oz (425 g) can	100	3.5	2.5	tr	100	0.25	–	9
Roe, cod's, 1 oz (30 g) fried	56	5.8	3.3	–	4.7	0.5	–	–
Roe, herring, fried, 1 oz (30 g)	68	5.9	4.4	–	4.5	0.5	–	–
Salad cream, 1 tablespoon	45	tr	4	–	5	tr	–	–
Salami, 1 oz (30 g)	137	5.4	12.6	–	2.8	0.28	–	–
Salmon, canned, 1 × 3½ oz (100 g) can	155	20	8	–	93	1.4	–	–
Sardines, canned, drained, 3½ oz (100 g)	217	23.7	13.6	–	550	2.9	–	–
Satsuma, 1	20	tr	tr	2	25	0.15	21	–
Sausagemeat, 1 oz (30 g)	102	2.9	9	–	11	0.3	–	–
Sausages:								
1 chipolata, well cooked	65	2.7	4.9	–	10	0.3	–	–
1 large, well cooked	120	5	9	–	20	0.6	–	–
1 large low-fat, well cooked	100	6	7	–	25	0.7	–	–

Scampi, deep-fried, 1 average serving, 5 oz (140 g)	450	17	24	–	138	1·5	–	–
Scone, 1, buttered	255	4	13·7	1·2	342	0·8	–	3
Shredded Wheat, 2	150	5	1·4	5·7	18	2	–	tr
Shrimp, shelled, 1 oz (30 g)	33	6·7	–	–	90	0·5	–	–
Skate, 1 wing, fried in batter, 6 oz (170 g)	350	31	21·	–	87	1·75	–	–
Soup, ½ pint, (300 ml):								
Cream of chicken	174	5·1	11·4	–	81	1·2	–	3·3
Cream of tomato	165	2·4	10	–	51	1·2	tr	78
Oxtail	132	7·2	5·1	–	120	3	–	2·7
Thick vegetable	111	4·5	2·1	varies	51	1·8	tr	7·5
Soya sauce, 1 tablespoon	13	tr	tr	–	n/k	0·75	–	tr
Spaghetti in tomato sauce, 1 × 7½ oz (213 g) can	140	3·6	1·5	–	45	0·86	tr	7·3
Spinach, 4 oz (115 g) serving	30	5	0·5	6·3	600	4	25	–
Sponge pudding, 4 oz (115 g) serving	340	5·9	16	1·2	210	1·2	tr	18
Sprats, fried, 4 oz (115 g)	385	22	33	–	620	4	–	–
Spring greens, 4 oz (115 g) serving	10	1·7	tr	3·8	86	1·3	30	–
Squash, orange, ½ pint (300 ml) made with 2 fl oz (60 ml) concentrate	70	–	–	–	5	tr	–	17
Strawberries, 4 oz (115 g) serving	26	0·6	tr	2·2	22	0·7	60	–
Suet, 1 oz (30 g)	230	tr	24	–	tr	tr	–	–
Suet pudding, 4 oz (115 g) serving	330	4·4	18	1·1	240	0·9	tr	14

Food	Calories	Protein (g)	Fat (g)	Fibre (g)	Calcium (mg)	Iron (mg)	Vitamin C (mg)	Added sugar (g)
Sugar, white or brown, 1 teaspoon	20	–	–	–	–	–	–	5
Sultanas, 1 oz (30 g)	71	tr	–	2	15	0·5	–	–
Swede, boiled, 4 oz (115 g) serving	18	1	tr	2·8	42	0·3	17	–
Sweet potato, baked or boiled, 4 oz (115 g)	85	1	0·6	2·3	21	0·6	15	–
Sweetcorn, boiled, 4 oz (115 g) serving	123	4	2·3	4·7	4	0·9	9	–
Syrup, golden, 1 tablespoon	45	tr	–	–	4	0·25	–	12
Taco shell, 1 × ⅓ oz (10·5 g)	50	1	2·5	0·75	n/k	n/k	–	n/k
Tangerine, 1	20	tr	tr	1·2	20	tr	18	–
Taramasalata, 1 tablespoon	70	1	7	–	4	tr	tr	–
Tartare sauce, 1 tablespoon	40	tr	3·2	–	n/k	n/k	–	n/k
Tea, black, 1 cup	1	tr	tr	–	tr	tr	–	–
Toffee, 1 oz (30 g)	120	0·5	4·7	–	26	0·42	–	20
Tomato, raw, 1	7	0·5	tr	0·75	7	0·2	10	–
Tomato juice, 4 fl oz (120 ml)	16	0·7	tr	–	10	0·5	20	–
Tomato ketchup, 1 tablespoon	14	0·3	tr	–	4	tr	–	5
Tomato purée, 1 tablespoon	10	0·9	tr	–	8	0·75	15	–
Tomatoes, canned, 1 small 7½ oz (215 g) can	25	2·3	tr	1·9	19	1·9	38	–
Tongue, 1 oz (30 g)	60	4·5	4·5	–	9	0·7	–	–
Tortilla chips, 1 × 5½ oz (150 g) bag	745	n/k	n/k	tr	n/k	n/k	–	–
Treacle, black, 1 tablespoon	38	tr	–	–	75	1·4	–	10

Treacle tart, average serving, 4 oz (115 g)	370	3·8	14	1·2	65	1·5	—	33
Trifle, 1 average serving, 4 oz (115 g)	160	3·5	6	—	82	0·7	1	18
Tripe, boiled, 4 oz (115 g) serving	100	14·8	4·5	—	150	0·7	3	—
Trout, cooked without fat, 1 average, 7 oz (200 g)	180	30	6	—	48	1·4	—	—
Tuna in oil, drained, 1 small (3½ oz, 100 g) can	215	25	12	—	7	1·1	—	—
Turkey, roast, lean, 1 oz (30 g) slice	40	8	1	—	3	0·25	—	—
Turkeyburger in breadcrumbs, average, dry-fried or grilled	220	10	10	—	10	0·5	—	—
Turnip, boiled, 4 oz (115 g)	14	0·7	tr	2·2	55	0·4	17	—
Vinegar, 1 tablespoon	0·5	tr	—	—	2·2	tr	—	—
Walnuts, shelled, 1 oz (30 g)	147	3	14	1·5	17	0·67	tr	—
Watercress, 1 oz (30 g)	4	0·8	tr	1	61	0·5	0·5	—
Weetabix, 2	130	4·4	1·3	4·9	13	2·9	—	2·3
White sauce, savoury, 4 oz (115 g) serving	150	4·3	10·3	—	140	0·3	—	—
Whitebait, deep-fried, average serving, 7 oz (200 g)	1,050	38	95	—	1,720	10·2	fr	—
Yogurt:								
Diet, fruit, 4½ oz (125 g) tub	50	5·1	0·1	tr	200	0·25	fr	—
Fruit, 4½ oz (125 g) tub	130	6	1·25	tr	200	0·25	2	17
Greek strained, 1 tablespoon	25	1	n/k	—	27	tr	fr	—

Food	Calories	Protein (g)	Fat (g)	Fibre (g)	Calcium (mg)	Iron (mg)	Vitamin C (mg)	Added sugar (g)
Natural, 1 tablespoon (low fat)	10	0·75	tr	–	27	tr	tr	–
Natural, 4½ oz (125 g) tub	80	6·25	1·25	–	225	tr	tr	–
Thick and Creamy, 4½ oz (125 g) tub	175	8·4	4·6	tr	200	0·25	2	17
Yorkshire pudding, 2 oz (55 g) serving	105	3·5	5	0·5	65	0·5	–	–

NOTE: All values are average and/or approximate

n/k = not known

tr = trace

FOR THE BEST IN PAPERBACKS, LOOK FOR THE

In every corner of the world, on every subject under the sun, Penguin represents quality and variety – the very best in publishing today.

For complete information about books available from Penguin – including Pelicans, Puffins, Peregrines and Penguin Classics – and how to order them, write to us at the appropriate address below. Please note that for copyright reasons the selection of books varies from country to country.

In the United Kingdom: Please write to *Dept E.P., Penguin Books Ltd, Harmondsworth, Middlesex, UB7 0DA*

In the United States: Please write to *Dept BA, Penguin, 299 Murray Hill Parkway, East Rutherford, New Jersey 07073*

In Canada: Please write to *Penguin Books Canada Ltd, 2801 John Street, Markham, Ontario L3R 1B4*

In Australia: Please write to the *Marketing Department, Penguin Books Australia Ltd, P.O. Box 257, Ringwood, Victoria 3134*

In New Zealand: Please write to the *Marketing Department, Penguin Books (NZ) Ltd, Private Bag, Takapuna, Auckland 9*

In India: Please write to *Penguin Overseas Ltd, 706 Eros Apartments, 56 Nehru Place, New Delhi, 110019*

In Holland: Please write to *Penguin Books Nederland B.V., Postbus 195, NL–1380AD Weesp, Netherlands*

In Germany: Please write to *Penguin Books Ltd, Friedrichstrasse 10–12, D–6000 Frankfurt Main 1, Federal Republic of Germany*

In Spain: Please write to *Longman Penguin España, Calle San Nicolas 15, E–28013 Madrid, Spain*

In France: Please write to *Penguin Books Ltd, 39 Rue de Montmorency, F-75003, Paris, France*

In Japan: Please write to *Longman Penguin Japan Co Ltd, Yamaguchi Building, 2–12–9 Kanda Jimbocho, Chiyoda-Ku, Tokyo 101, Japan*

FOR THE BEST IN PAPERBACKS, LOOK FOR THE

COOKERY IN PENGUINS

The Beginner's Cookery Book   Betty Falk

Revised and updated, this book is for aspiring cooks of all ages who want to make appetizing and interesting meals without too much fuss. With an emphasis on healthy eating, this is the ideal starting point for would-be cooks.

The Pleasure of Vegetables   Elisabeth Ayrton

'Every dish in this beautifully written book seems possible to make and gorgeous to eat' – *Good Housekeeping*

French Provincial Cooking   Elizabeth David

'One could cook for a lifetime on this book alone' – *Observer*

Jane Grigson's Fruit Book

Fruit is colourful, refreshing and life-enhancing; this book shows how it can also be absolutely delicious in meringues or compotes, soups or pies.

A Taste of American Food   Clare Walker

Far from being just a junk food culture, American cuisine is the most diverse in the world. Swedish, Jewish, Creole and countless other kinds of food have been adapted to the new environment; this book gives some of the most delicious recipes.

Leaves from Our Tuscan Kitchen   Janet Ross and Michael Waterfield

A revised and updated version of a great cookery classic, this splendid book contains some of the most unusual and tasty vegetable recipes in the world.

COOKERY IN PENGUINS

Simple French Food   Richard Olney

'There is no other book about food that is anything like it . . . essential and exciting reading for cooks, of course, but it is also a book for eaters . . . its pages brim over with invention' – Paul Levy in the *Observer*

The Vegetarian Epicure   Anna Thomas

Mouthwatering recipes for soups, breads, vegetable dishes, salads and desserts that any meat-eater or vegetarian will find hard to resist.

A Book of Latin American Cooking   Elisabeth Lambert Ortiz

Anyone who thinks Latin American food offers nothing but *tacos* and *tortillas* will enjoy the subtle marriages of texture and flavour celebrated in this marvellous guide to one of the world's most colourful *cuisines*.

Quick Cook   Beryl Downing

For victims of the twentieth century, this book provides some astonishing gourmet meals – all cooked in under thirty minutes.

Josceline Dimbleby's Book of Puddings, Desserts and Savouries

'Full of the most delicious and novel ideas for every type of pudding' – *Lady*

Chinese Food   Kenneth Lo

A popular step-by-step guide to the whole range of delights offered by Chinese cookery and the fascinating philosophy behind it.

COOKERY IN PENGUINS

Fast Food for Vegetarians   Janette Marshall

Packed with ideas for healthy, delicious dishes from Caribbean vegetables to rose-water baklava, this stimulating book proves that fast food does not have to mean junk food.

More Easy Cooking for One or Two   Louise Davies

This charming book, full of ideas and easy recipes, offers even the novice cook good wholesome food with the minimum of effort.

The Cuisine of the Rose   Mireille Johnston

Classic French cooking from Burgundy and Lyonnais, including the most succulent dishes of meat and fish bathed in pungent sauces of wine and herbs.

Good Food from Your Freezer   Helge Rubinstein and Sheila Bush

Using a freezer saves endless time and trouble and cuts your food bills dramatically; this book will enable you to cook just as well – perhaps even better – with a freezer as without.

Roy Ackerman's Recipe Collection

Here is a treasure-trove of recipes that have been created by some of the top chefs in the very best restaurants in the British Isles. Handwritten and beautifully illustrated, it is a stunning selection of their favourite dishes, gathered together to recreate memories of a special experience.

Budget Gourmet   Geraldene Holt

Plan carefully, shop wisely and cook well to produce first-rate food at minimal expense. It's as easy as pie!

The Prime of Your Life   Dr Miriam Stoppard

The first comprehensive, fully illustrated guide to healthy living for people aged fifty and beyond, by top medical writer and media personality, Dr Miriam Stoppard.

A Good Start   Louise Graham

Factual and practical, full of tips on providing a healthy and balanced diet for young children, *A Good Start* is essential reading for all parents.

How to Get Off Drugs   Ira Mothner and Alan Weitz

This book is a vital contribution towards combating drug addiction in Britain in the eighties. For drug abusers, their families and their friends.

Naturebirth   Danaë Brook

A pioneering work which includes suggestions on diet and health, exercises and many tips on the 'natural' way to prepare for giving birth in a joyful relaxed way.

Pregnancy   Dr Jonathan Scher and Carol Dix

Containing the most up-to-date information on pregnancy – the effects of stress, sexual intercourse, drugs, diet, late maternity and genetic disorders – this book is an invaluable and reassuring guide for prospective parents.

Care of the Dying   Richard Lamerton

It is never true that 'nothing more can be done' for the dying. This book shows us how to face death without pain, with humanity, with dignity and in peace.

FOR THE BEST IN PAPERBACKS, LOOK FOR THE ⓟ

PENGUIN HEALTH

Medicines: A Guide for Everybody   Peter Parish

This sixth edition of a comprehensive survey of all the medicines available over the counter or on prescription offers clear guidance for the ordinary reader as well as invaluable information for those involved in health care.

Pregnancy and Childbirth   Sheila Kitzinger

A complete and up-to-date guide to physical and emotional preparation for pregnancy – a must for all prospective parents.

The Penguin Encyclopaedia of Nutrition   John Yudkin

This book cuts through all the myths about food and diets to present the real facts clearly and simply. 'Everyone should buy one' – *Nutrition News and Notes*

The Parents' A to Z   Penelope Leach

For anyone with a child of 6 months, 6 years or 16 years, this guide to all the little problems involved in their health, growth and happiness will prove reassuring and helpful.

Jane Fonda's Workout Book

Help yourself to better looks, superb fitness and a whole new approach to health and beauty with this world-famous and fully illustrated programme of diet and exercise advice.

Alternative Medicine   Andrew Stanway

Dr Stanway provides an objective and practical guide to thirty-two alternative forms of therapy – from Acupuncture and the Alexander Technique to Macrobiotics and Yoga.